Harnessing Official Statistics

Edited by
Deana Leadbeter

Radcliffe Medical Press

Radcliffe Medical Press
18 Marcham Road, Abingdon, Oxon OX14 1AA

British Library Cataloguing in Publication Data

A catalogue record for this book is available from the British Library.

ISBN 1 85775 354 2

Typeset by Joshua Associates Ltd, Oxford
Printed and bound by TJ International Ltd, Padstow, Cornwall

Contents

Series Editor's Preface

Harnessing Official Statistics

Whenever those entering the world of statistical analysis of health-care wish to position their own local findings or expectations, they naturally think of looking to nationally produced data analyses. However, they will soon discover that official statistics are difficult for the beginner to understand and to find their way around. Not only are there a number of official bodies, including the Office for National Statistics (ONS), the Department of Health and the NHS Executive, but there are also recognised agencies such as the UK Data Archive and the National Centre for Health Outcomes Development. New entrants to this world are not the only ones to find themselves confused or afraid that they have missed an important aspect.

This specially commissioned addition to the *Harnessing Health Information Series* aims to meet this need, by helping readers through the important function of *Harnessing Official Statistics*. It takes the reader systematically through the statistical functions and outputs of the key organisations and programmes. It does not merely list published data analyses, but by giving the background and methods of each official statistical function it highlights strengths and relevance to particular uses.

Organisational domains are covered including hospital statistics and the fast-moving area of primary care. Subsequent chapters then consider particular application areas including maternal and child health statistical systems and cancer registry processes. Dedicated chapters address outcomes studies, and use of health survey data. Concluding chapters look at cross-sectoral data linkage, and consider future statistical development needs.

This volume has been assembled and edited by Deana Leadbeter, who as Chair of the Health Statistics User Group is ideally placed to see the subject from both statistics user and statistics provider viewpoints. Thanks to her contacts and knowledge of the scene, each chapter is contributed by a top subject expert and full co-operation has been forthcoming from official bodies.

Harnessing Health Information has many aspects and official statistics have an essential, but often under-exploited, contribution to make. It is hoped that this volume on *Harnessing Official Statistics* meets the objective of making official statistics more widely understood and accessible.

Michael Rigby
August 2000

About the authors

Sheila Anderson BA MA is the Director of Depositor Services at The Data Archive, University of Essex, the national social science archive for the UK. She studied sociology and social history at the University of Essex where she developed an interest in the use of digital resources for research. Following a spell working as a researcher at the Cambridge Group for the History of Population and Social Structure, she moved back to the University of Essex to work at The Data Archive. For the last 10 years, she has been actively involved in acquiring and managing social science and historical data resources for use in research and teaching, including key resources for health-related research.

Madhavi Bajekal PhD is a senior researcher at the National Centre for Social Research. She completed her PhD in economic history at the University of London in 1991 and joined the Department of Population Sciences and General Practice at Imperial College, London, where she continues to hold an Honorary Research Fellowship. Dr Bajekal has undertaken a range of health-related research, focusing primarily on health needs assessment and resource allocation for primary care. At the National Centre, she is a member of the team which carried out the 1999 *Health Survey for England*, which focused on the health of black, Irish and minority ethnic groups. She is seconded to the Department of Health on a part-time basis to provide research and health information support.

John Charlton MSc DIC HonMFPHM is currently Principal Methodologist in the Office for National Statistics, having begun his public health career as lecturer in medical statistics at the Department of Public Health Medicine, United Medical and Dental Schools of Guy's and St Thomas's Hospitals. He subsequently worked for the Department of Health before joining the Office for National Statistics. His research outputs include developing avoidable mortality outcome indicators, suicide, disability and resource allocation. He has worked with GP, hospital and mortality data, and was responsible for the statistical aspects of the *Fourth National GP Morbidity Survey*. Recently, he was editor and contributed to two ONS decennial volumes on *The Health of Adult Britain*.

Colin Cryer BSc PhD CStat HonMFPHM is statistician and injury research team leader at the Centre for Health Service Studies at Tunbridge Wells, University of Kent. He gained his BSc in Applied Mathematics and Statistics, and his PhD in Statistics, at University College of Wales Aberystwyth. He spent five years working for a pharmaceutical company supporting the development of medicines, and 10 years teaching statistics in a medical school in New Zealand, prior to his current position. His present interests include the identification of risk factors for, and the prevention of, falls in older people, the use of data linkage to facilitate injury prevention, and the use of routine data sources for monitoring the occurrence of non-fatal injury.

Vic Kempner DipHSM MHSM MIMgt is Acting Head of the London IMT Unit, a collaboratively funded group working for the 16 local health communities in London. He has wide experience of health statistics and information in a variety of NHS organisations, having been a user of data whilst working in planning and general management posts, as well as a supplier of it in various information service roles.

Azim Lakhani MA BMBCh FFPHM is Director of the National Centre for Health Outcomes Development, based jointly at the London School of Hygiene and Tropical Medicine, University of London and at the Institute of Health Sciences, University of Oxford. Following undergraduate medical training at Oxford University, he undertook post-graduate training in public health medicine and is now an accredited specialist. He was previously Director of Public Health in West Lambeth Health Authority, and more recently Director of the Central Health Outcomes Unit within the government Department of Health. In addition, he has been involved in voluntary work on social development and poverty alleviation with the Aga Khan Development Network, the World Faiths Development Dialogue and the World Bank.

Deana Leadbeter BSc MSc is an international health information specialist at the Centre for Health Service Studies at Tunbridge Wells, University of Kent, and is also currently Centre Co-ordinator for the Professional Awards in IM&T (Health) at the Salomons Centre, Canterbury Christ Church University College. She worked as a statistician in pharmaceutical research before joining the NHS as

Regional Statistician for the South East Thames Regional Health Authority, and then moving to the South East Institute of Public Health as Director of Information Services. She is involved in a variety of health information projects, both nationally and internationally, working with local teams to understand the information required to support the health system, and to specify, implement and use the information systems needed. She currently chairs the UK Health Statistics User Group.

Alison Macfarlane BA DipStat CStat HonMFPHM worked as a statistician on a variety of subjects, including animal husbandry, transportation planning, the health effects of air pollution and child health before joining the National Perinatal Epidemiology Unit when it was founded in 1978. Much of her work there has been on the interpretation and use of routine statistics and she is co-author (with Miranda Mugford) of two editions of *Birth Counts: statistics of pregnancy and childbirth*. She has also been involved in research on place of birth, and a national study of triplet and higher order births.

Gillian Matthews BA FRCOG FFPHM is a former Regional Health Authority Consultant in Public Health Medicine and was subsequently Acting Director of the Thames Cancer Registry. For many years she used clinical and service data as the foundation of her work in health service development. At Thames Cancer Registry she had operational responsibility for the development of information systems, and production of management and outcome data covering malignant disease in the 14 million population of South-East England.

Steve Price has been employed within the statistics division of the Department of Health since 1994, having previously held a variety of posts at the Department of Social Security. Throughout this time he has assisted in the operation and further development of the Hospital Episode Statistics (HES) System, and in the training of staff needing access to the system. Steve has also taken a lead in the development of the new HES publications strategy, which has included the provision of summary in-patient data via the Internet.

1 Introduction

Deana Leadbeter

The topic of this book is *Harnessing Official Statistics* and it is concerned with official statistics in relation to health and healthcare. Decisions about health and healthcare, whether made by policy makers, by health professionals or by the public, are influenced by the information that is available. Much of this information is derived from official statistics and, in many cases, is made available through the Government Statistical Service. The quality and accessibility of official statistics can therefore have a major influence on our ability to monitor health and healthcare.

Definition of official statistics

In the consultation document *Statistics: a matter of trust*, published by HM Treasury in 1998,[1] there was a move away from the use of the term official statistics to the concept of 'national statistics', to cover all work supporting the production of statistics intended for public use. This broadening of the definition has been welcomed by the health statistics user community, and is the interpretation taken in this book. The definition could perhaps even be broadened further to cover all NHS statistics, and to include information about health and social care provided in the private sector, whether publicly or privately funded.

Following the consultation, a White Paper *Building Trust in Statistics*[2] has been issued which proposes the setting up of a Statistics Commission which would oversee the production and use of official or national statistics. It is not clear at the time of writing what effect this White Paper will have on the collection and availability of statistics relevant to the health service. A Head of National Statistics (to be referred to as the National Statistician) will be appointed and a Framework for National Statistics will be published which will set out detailed roles and responsibilities. It is expected that information on this will be available through the various government websites. Useful sites to find out the current position on this, and on other issues in relation to official statistics are http://www.open.gov.uk/, http://www.statistics.gov.uk/, and http://www.ons.gov.uk/. Websites relating specifically to health or health services information are the Department of Health's site, http://www.doh.gov.uk/, and the website of the NHS Information Authority, http://www.nhsia.nhs.uk/.

The White Paper notes that there are three ways of defining national statistics – in terms of the people providing the service, the activities or the outputs. In the first instance the scope of National Statistics will be defined by outputs and will only cover current Office for National Statistics publications and public access databases. However other statistics published by government departments can be included with the agreement of Ministers. It is also recognised within the White Paper that some respondents to the consultation favoured extending this coverage and so the government will ask the Statistics Commission to keep the scope of National Statistics under review.

This is just one example of where changes are underway that may affect the data collected and the information available. In fact, many of the areas mentioned in this book are currently under review. For example, birth and death statistics, which are mentioned in Chapters 2, 9 and 10, are collected by registrars of births and deaths (RBDs) throughout England and Wales. This system was reviewed during 1999, since it was felt that the current structure of the registration system, and outdated legislation, no longer provide a service appropriate to the modern day. The consultation so far on this review has indicated that there is a demand for a flexible range of statistical information derived from the civil registration system, and the information currently collected does not satisfy requirements.

If changes are recommended they are likely to take some time to be introduced and it is expected that they will be widely publicised via the various official statistics websites. However, users of official statistics should be aware that many information systems are continually under review and they should check the current position before commencing any work. Wherever possible, in the following chapters, websites or contact names are given, from whence further information can be obtained.

Scope of this book

Even though the broad definition of official statistics is the one being used, it is not possible within this book to discuss how to access and use all possible sources of information relevant to the health sector that have been produced for public use. The approach that has therefore been followed has been to cover some of the major data sources and then to look at selected areas in more detail. These topic areas have been selected both because they are important in terms of health, and because they illustrate approaches that need to be taken when accessing and using data from official sources.

Chapters 2, 3 and 4 cover the data available from the Office for National Statistics (ONS) and from the Department of Health (DoH)'s Hospital Episode Statistics (HES) database, and Chapter 12 looks at aggregated data from statistical returns. Since much of the data routinely available on health services activity relates to secondary care, Chapter 5 considers information from a primary care perspective. Chapter 7 looks in detail at the Health Survey for England and illustrates how official health surveys carried out at national level can be used both for national policy development and also at a more local level.

Health and healthcare information in relation to three specific areas – maternity, cancer and injury – are considered in more detail in Chapters 9, 10 and 11. As has already been mentioned, these three areas have been selected to illustrate the approaches that need to be taken when considering an area in detail, and are not intended to provide complete coverage of all areas of health service statistics. Chapter 9 looks at maternity statistics and also serves to illustrate how different data sources, and issues in relation to availability, deficiencies and data quality, need to be considered when investigating a particular area in more detail. Chapter 10 covers the role of cancer registries in supporting the work of the NHS. Chapter 11 looks at injury data, and also provides an example of data linkage between NHS and non-NHS datasets.

As well as information provided directly by data producers, access to relevant data can be provided by the Economics and Social Research Council (ESRC) Data Archive, which is housed at the University of Essex. This Archive houses the largest collection of accessible computer readable data in the social sciences and humanities in the UK and this is discussed further in Chapter 6. Another national archive, which is not discussed in detail in this book, is the National Digital Archive of Datasets (NDAD). This contains archived digital data from UK government departments and agencies. The system has been available since March 1998 and at present only has a limited amount of health data available, although this may increase in future. It provides open access to the catalogues of all its holdings, and free access to open datasets following a simple registration process. Further information can be obtained from http://ndad.ulcc.ac.uk/.

Finally, in Chapter 8, there is a review of recent work by the Centre for Health Outcomes on bringing together, and rationalising, all current and planned health-related indicators.

These chapters do not cover all possible sources and uses of official statistics. However, the aim is to give an indication of how to identify available sources of relevant data, even if they are not specifically mentioned in this book, and to highlight the issues that need to be considered when accessing and using such data.

National coverage

There are differences between the four countries of the UK in the way health and social services statistics are compiled which often make it difficult to compile statistics for the UK as a whole. It is hoped that, when the Statistics Commission is appointed, it will be answerable to the devolved bodies in Wales, Scotland and Northern Ireland as well as to the UK Parliament, and will work with statistical bodies in each country to promote harmonisation. In the White Paper it states that the Statistics Commission will report to the UK Parliament and that 'the devolved administrations will subsequently wish to consider the working relationships they wish to establish with the Commission'.

Users of official statistics need to be aware that differences exist between the four countries in both terminology and in the data items collected. For example, although the emphasis on a primary care-led health service is the same across all four countries, in England there are primary care groups and trusts, whereas in Wales there are local care groups, in Scotland there are primary care trusts and local care cooperatives, and in Northern Ireland there are health and social care partnerships.

It has not been possible within this book to look at each country separately. Wherever possible reference has been to the UK as a whole, and differences between the four countries in the data collected and the information available have been highlighted. However in some chapters the focus is primarily on the situation in England. Further information on the situation in the individual countries can be obtained from the relevant websites: for the Northern Ireland Office http://www.nics.gov.uk/, for the Scottish Office http://www.scotland.gov.uk/, and for the Welsh Office http://www.wales.gov.uk/welcome.html.

Meeting the needs of different users

The review by Sir Derek Rayner in the early 1980s concluded that statistical information should be primarily collected to satisfy the needs of government, which led to a reduced service from the Government Statistical Service (GSS) during the 1980s. However this view subsequently changed, as evidenced by the White Paper on Open Government in 1993,[3] and, more recently, the consultation paper on Official Statistics mentioned above.[1,2] The background to these and subsequent developments on access to information is given in a series of *Your Right to Know* guidance notes produced by the Home Office.[4] The current view of the GSS, and of most other producers of official statistics, is that the statistics are produced to serve not only government but also the wider community.

The members of the wider community of health statistics users come from different organisational backgrounds, including Parliament, government departments, health service organisations, researchers, voluntary organisations, and the public. These users may have very different levels of expertise. They will include experienced users who may require access to data to carry out their own analyses, regular users of statistical summaries and other analyses carried out centrally, users wishing to access information via the Web, and users with no computing facilities or expertise who wish to access the information on paper in libraries.

Increasingly producers of official statistics are making the information they produce available in different formats and through different mechanisms to suit the differing needs of the user community. Users of official statistics should check with the data producers on the options currently available. The levels of expertise that users have may vary depending on the data being accessed. Experienced users may wish to class themselves as inexperienced in relation to data with which they are less familiar, and so access these data through a route that provides more support or advice.

Using the Internet

Both changes in policy and developments in information technology (IT) can affect not only the data collected but also the mechanism whereby the information can be accessed and used. The fact that some of the references given, in this chapter and elsewhere in the book, are in terms of websites is something that would not have been commonplace only a few years ago. The widespread use of the Internet has meant that this is now used as a common method of disseminating information about statistics, as well as providing access to the actual data in some cases. As is mentioned in Chapter 2, information on UK publications and data can now be found on STATBASE (http://www.statistics.gov.uk). This is only a relatively recent development and it is expected that the amount of information provided through this route will increase. It is made up of two components: StatSearch, a free electronic catalogue listing all the latest Government Statistical Service products, and StatStore, a database of key economic and social statistics, mostly available free of charge, with more detailed data available on a chargeable basis.

One of the problems that users can find when trying to obtain information via the Web is identifying relevant and reliable information on the topic of interest amongst the many millions of pages available on the Web. A useful introduction to finding health information on the Web is Robert Kiley's book *The Doctor's Internet Handbook*.[5] One point he makes is that the best route to finding statistical information is often to consider first which organisation is likely to publish this type of information. This principle applies whether the search for information is via the Web or via telephone contact or via a library. A more general explanation of the Internet and its use in healthcare can be found in an earlier book in the *Harnessing Health Information* series.[6]

Using a narrow definition of official statistics for the health sector, the relevant organisations would just be the Office for National Statistics (ONS) and the Department of Health (DoH). Although these are still very important producers of health statistics, the use of the broader definition of national statistics means that there are many other organisations that produce statistics relevant to the health sector, that are intended for public use. Non–NHS data sources are discussed further below.

Data quality

It is essential that users of official statistics fully understand any quality issues relating to these data, if they are to interpret them correctly. Increasingly, data producers are aiming to produce data quality information with the data they provide. Users should be made aware of:

- data quality and completeness
- any validation and audit carried out, and whether this has resulted in any amendments being made to the data
- clear definitions of the data items plus, ideally, some comments on what the data items measure. It is impossible to anticipate all the purposes for which data might be used once they have been published, and this makes it crucial to document what they do actually measure
- fitness of information outputs for the various uses to which they may be put.

Users of official statistics should contact the data producers if they feel they have not been given sufficient information on quality issues.

Non-NHS data sources

It is important to be able to access non–NHS data when looking at health needs, since the determinants of health often lie outside the health service. Work in relation to prevention of illness and the promotion of good health therefore requires access to data from a wide range of sources. There is also an increasing emphasis within the health sector on partnership working with other agencies, and the need to share information on common and related issues. Health and healthcare activities can be affected by activities in other sectors, and monitoring and planning of health services' activity need to take this into account.

A guide to data sources to help people working in public health in London, within and outside the NHS, has been produced by the

Health of Londoners' project.[7] Although some of these sources are specific to London, many of the sources mentioned are of relevance generally. This document is available on the Health of Londoners' website, www.elcha.co.uk/holp/, and it is intended that it will be updated by users on an ongoing basis. Further details can be obtained from David Morgan on davidm@elcha.co.uk.

Some of the main sources are summarised below. The interpretation of information available from some of these official sources is discussed in *Interpreting Official Statistics*, edited by Ruth Levitas and Will Guy,[8] and in *Statistics in Society: the arithmetic of politics*, edited by Daniel Dorling and Stephen Simpson.[9] The first of these books examines the official statistics produced about the current state of British society and discusses what can be learned from the available data. This includes a chapter on measuring health and on health inequality. The second discusses how social statistics, including those concerning health and healthcare, are used to make decisions in our society. A fuller account of the sources of particular interest to the health sector is given in *Official Health Statistics: an unofficial guide*.[10]

There are also currently several Statistics User Groups that carry out activities to support the use of statistics in their particular areas. A list of these groups, together with current ONS Advisory Groups, is given in the ONS publication *Official Statistics: governance and consultation*.[11]

Non-NHS data sources include population estimates, vital statistics, and census data which are covered in Chapters 2 and 3. Interpretation of much of these and other data depends on grouping into geographical areas. There may be different administrative geographies for different purposes and these may not all be co-terminous. This issue is discussed with respect to London in David Morgan's paper mentioned above.

Various deprivation indices, some of which are derived from the Census, are used when analysing and interpreting data relating to the health sector. Indices developed by Townsend and also by Carstairs are widely used,[12,13] as are Jarman's Under Privileged Areas (UPA) scores which are based on a survey of GPs.[14,15,16] The Department of Environment Index of Local Conditions is widely used by local government. Work was underway to produce a new version of this index in 1999. Progress with this project is given on http://index99.apsoc.ox.ac.uk/.

In addition to these indices there are indices developed as part of the NHS resource allocation process. The most recent indices are based on work by the University of York, which was commissioned by the NHS Executive.[17] The resource allocation formula is kept under continuous review, and guidance on the current formulae is issued in Health Service Circulars.[18]

The UK publishes two measures of unemployment: one is an administrative measure called the claimant count and the other measure comes from the Labour Force Survey. Full details of all labour market-related statistical outputs and products can be accessed through the ONS website (http://www.statistics.gov.uk). Claimant counts by parliamentary constituency are published every month as a research paper by the House of Commons Library. Data are available to the general public through the House of Commons Library website (http://www.parliament.uk/commons/lib/research/). The Department for Education and Employment (DfEE)'s website is http://www.dfee.gov.uk .

The general website for the Houses of Parliament is also a useful source for a range of statistical information that may be contained in Hansard or in the proceedings of Select Committees. Enquiries can also be made to the House of Commons Information Office (020 7219 4272 or hcinfo@parliament.uk).

Accessing comprehensive information on income can be difficult, but there are a number of national surveys that collect income information including the Family Resources Survey, Labour Force Survey, New Earnings Survey, and General Household Survey. There is also an annual statistical series, Households Below Average Income (HBAI). Further information on this can be obtained from the Department of Social Security website (http:/www.dss.gov.uk). Information about benefits can be obtained from the Local Government Management Board (contact emma.jenkins@lgmb.gov.uk).

Use of police data on accidents is discussed in Chapter 11. Summary details of the British Crime Survey, and also prison population data, are available from the Home Office website (http://www.homeoffice.gov.uk).

The links between housing and health have been well established. Some data are available from the Census, and information about housing stock can be obtained from local authority Housing Improvement Programme (HIP) submissions. Poor air quality is also considered to be detrimental to health. Details of the National

Air Quality Strategy (consultation document published in January 1999), and also regularly updated air quality bulletins, are available from the Department of the Environment, Transport and the Regions (DETR) website (http://www.detr.gov.uk/).

As with the NHS data mentioned above this is not a comprehensive list of non-NHS sources, but it indicates some of the information available for a few of the main factors that can affect health. Official statistics cover a wide range of areas, and many of these need to be considered when accessing and using official statistics to maintain and improve health and healthcare for the UK population.

References

1 HM Treasury (1998) *Statistics: a matter of trust – a consultation document.* Cmd 3882. The Stationery Office, London.
2 HM Treasury (1999) *Building Trust in Statistics.* Cmd 4412. The Stationery Office, London.
3 Home Office (1993) *Open Government.* Cmd 2290. The Stationery Office, London.
4 Home Office (1999) *'Your Right to Know' guidance notes.* Available on http://www.homeoffice.gov.uk/foi/ or from Freedom of Information Unit, Home Office, 50 Queen Anne's Gate, London.
5 Kiley R (1998) *The Doctor's Internet Handbook.* The Royal Society of Medicine Press Limited, London.
6 Tyrrell S (1999) *Using the Internet in Healthcare.* Radcliffe Medical Press, Oxford.
7 Morgan D and Bardsley M (1999) *Non NHS Data Relevant to Health: a guide to sources.* Health of Londoners' project, Department of Public Health, East London and the City Health Authority. Available at www.elcha.co.uk/holp/.
8 Levitas R and Guy W (eds) (1996) *Interpreting Official Statistics.* Routledge, London.
9 Dorling D and Simpson S (eds) (1999) *Statistics in Society: the arithmetic of politics.* Arnold, London.
10 Kerrison SH and Macfarlane A (1999) *Official Health Statistics: an unofficial guide.* Arnold, London.
11 ONS (published annually) *Official Statistics: governance and consultation.* Office for National Statistics, London.
12 Carstairs V and Morris R (1989) Deprivation and mortality: an alternative to social class? *Community Medicine.* **11**: 210–19.

13 Townsend P, Phillimore P and Beattie A (1988) *Health and Deprivation: inequality and the North?* Croom Helm, London.

14 Jarman B (1983) Identification of underprivileged areas. *British Medical Journal.* **286**: 1705–8.

15 Jarman B (1984) Underprivileged areas: validation and distribution of scores. *British Medical Journal.* **289**: 1587–92.

16 Dolan SA, Jarman B, Bajekal M *et al.* (1995) Measuring disadvantage: changes in the under privileged, Townsend and Carstairs scores between 1981 and 1991. *Journal of Epidemiology and Community Health.* **49**: S30–3.

17 Carr-Hill RA, Hardman G, Martin S *et al.* (1994) *A Formula for Distributing NHS Revenues Based on Small Area Use of Hospital Beds.* Centre for Health Economics, University of York, York.

18 NHS Executive (1998) *The New NHS: modern, dependable – guidance on health authority and primary care allocations.* Health Service Circular HSC 1998/171. NHSE, Leeds.

2 ONS data: mortality

John Charlton

Introduction

This chapter, and the next, review the routine data available for monitoring the health of the UK population for which the Office for National Statistics (ONS) is responsible, including births, deaths, censuses and surveys. They briefly describe some of the analyses carried out within the ONS for government use and other clients, and how such data are made available to non-ONS users. Although focusing on England and Wales, comparisons are made with other parts of Britain. Detailed and up to date information on UK government publications and data can be found on STATBASE (http://www.statistics.gov.uk).

The most absolute measure of adverse health is death, and mortality data have been collected nationally since 1837. Death rates have traditionally been used as crude, but often effective, surrogates for more comprehensive measures of disease. This is often justified by the fact that death is unambiguous and the data collection is complete. However, use of mortality data alone could provide misleading impressions of the burdens of disease in society. For example, musculoskeletal disorders (including rheumatism and arthritis) are the most important current causes of limiting long-standing illness[1] but one of the least prevalent causes of death. Health service records provide a great deal of health-related data but are strongly influenced by variations in access to healthcare and patient help-seeking behaviour. Additionally, doctors treating sick and dying people are often only aware of the disease presented to them. Apart from this there is a large 'iceberg of disease'[2] that is not brought to the medical profession's attention. This includes diseases such as hypertension that have not yet caused symptoms, and problems that patients have chosen not to present to their doctor for one reason or another. General practitioners may also not be aware of disabilities encountered by their patients. A variety of studies are required in order to learn about health problems independently of service utilisation factors. These include screening studies with standardised procedures to detect unidentified as well as identified disease levels in the population. Community surveys are needed to elicit information on disability levels, self rating of health and subjective experiences of health or its absence. 'Lifestyle', which describes choices about food, smoking, drinking, how leisure time is spent, and social behaviour, can only be measured via surveys. Sometimes health-related behaviours which are likely to lead to ill-health, such as smoking, drinking and illicit drug use, are monitored as proxy health measures. It is also important to collect and analyse trend data on environmental aspects that are suspected of influencing health status or known to do so, such as: poverty; diet; employment conditions; education; housing; social isolation; genetic inheritance; transport; and environmental pollution. Non-mortality sources of health data are covered in Chapter 3.

Availability of mortality data

Although some data on numbers of deaths and their causes first became available from the weekly London Bills of Mortality which began in 1532, they were not complete, and the terms used were often inexact. The Births and Deaths Registration Act, which took effect from 1 July 1837, provided for the registration of every death which occurred in England and Wales, with a space in the prescribed register for the cause of death. The General Register Office (later to become Office of Population, Censuses and Surveys (OPCS) and subsequently Office for National Statistics (ONS)) was established in order to carry out the requirements of the Act. Registration of deaths in Scotland began with the Registration of Births, Deaths and Marriages (Scotland) Act of 1854. In 1839 William Farr introduced the first classification of causes of death, published in the Registrar General's first report.

Mortality data for England and Wales became comprehensive from 1841 onwards. In the same year the Registrar General conducted the national population census for the first time, which formed a sounder basis for population estimates than previous censuses. Censuses have been undertaken at 10-year intervals since then (except in 1941), and provide reliable denominators from which mortality rates can be calculated. ONS has published mortality trends since 1841,[3,4] and data are available on CD-ROM from 1901 onwards, classified by age, sex, and detailed cause. Confidential socio-economic information is obtained at the time of death registration on a draft entry form (Form 310) and is used by the ONS and General Register Office (Scotland) for statistical analyses.[4]

Factors likely to affect interpretation

Mortality trends by cause could reflect variations in disease incidence, case fatality rates or statistical artefacts.[5] Care needs to be taken in using mortality data to examine health trends. The way that diseases have been described and classified has varied over time, affecting the interpretation (*see* Table 2.1).

Completeness of data

In the earlier years of death registration the accuracy of certification was well below the standards we would find acceptable today, and it is also likely that some deaths were not registered.[6] There was no penalty for failure to register. The onus of registration was placed on the registrar rather than the informant, who could only be prosecuted if he/she refused to give information after being asked to do so by the registrar. Incomplete death registration was less of a problem than birth registration because bodies could only legally be buried after registration. The 1836 Act did not require that the cause of death be obtained from a medical practitioner, and medical services were expensive, which was another cause of inaccuracy. Additionally many doctors certifying deaths would have been trained in the late eighteenth and early nineteenth centuries, when medical knowledge was limited. Some of the causes of death described in the early tables published by the Registrar General seem somewhat bizarre today; for example a small 'epidemic' of 22 deaths from 'tight boots' occurred between 1894 and 1900 – a cause of death that has not been described at any other time.

Accuracy of data

In 1874 a new law, the Births and Deaths Registration Act, led to an improvement in the accuracy of death certification. It placed a duty on the medical practitioners attendant during the person's last illness to provide a cause of death, unless an inquest was being held, in which case the coroner's verdict was recorded. A penalty was introduced if the death was not registered. It also improved the quality of certification for infants and stillborn children. However, even then not all deaths were in fact certified by qualified medical practitioners. In 1879, 5% of deaths were still not certified in this way, although by 1928 this proportion had fallen to 1%.[3] In 1926 an Act made it unlawful to dispose of a body of a dead person before a registrar's certificate or coroner's order had been issued, and also required the registration of stillbirths.

Nowadays few if any deaths escape registration, and the cause of almost every registered death has been certified by a medical practitioner or coroner. All deaths must be registered with a Registrar of Births and Deaths, usually within five days in England and Wales or eight days in Scotland. In order to do this a medical certificate of cause of death is required, usually signed by the medical practitioner who attended the deceased during his/her last illness. With sudden death, suspected unnatural death or suspected industrial disease, the case will be referred to a coroner in England and Wales or to the Procurator Fiscal in Scotland, who will certify the death, possibly after holding a post mortem and/or inquest (see Figure 2.1). Coding of the underlying cause (see later) follows rules laid down by the World Health Organization.[7]

Changes in coding system

The way in which the descriptions on death certificates have been coded has varied. Farr's 1839 classification of cause of death was changed in 1881 and again in 1901. The second International Classification of Diseases (ICD) was adopted by the Registrar General in 1911. The international classification has subsequently been revised approximately every 10 years, to keep pace with advances in medical knowledge, and incidence of 'new' diseases. The tenth revision (ICD10) has been in use in the NHS since 1995, but cause of death is still coded to the ninth revision. The ONS plans to implement ICD10 for mortality data in England and Wales from January 2001 using coding software developed in the USA by the National Center for Health Statistics.

ICD10 will give a more up to date classification of causes of death, in line with current concepts. However, the change will cause difficulties in interpreting time trends. The main issue in mortality coding is not the codes for individual conditions, but the rules used to select a single underlying cause of death from all the conditions

Table 2.1 Factors which may have affected recorded mortality by cause

1532	London Bills of Mortality, some towns, parish records – incomplete picture of mortality.
1837	The Births and Deaths Registration Act of 1836, operationalised 1 July 1837, comprehensive registration data for deaths in England and Wales from 1841 onwards. But no penalty for failure to register, and doctors need not provide cause details.
1874	The Births and Deaths Registration Act of 1874 required the medical practitioners who were attendant during the person's last illness to provide a cause of death unless an inquest was being held. A penalty was introduced if the death was not registered. Also improved the quality of certification for infants and stillborn children.
1881	Changes to classification of causes of death.
1901	Changes to classification of causes of death. ONS used a variant of the first International Classification of Diseases (ICD1).★
1911	Adoption of the 2nd ICD revision (ICD2).★★
1921	Adoption of the 3rd ICD revision (ICD3).★★
1926	1926 Act made it unlawful to dispose of a body of a dead person before a registrar's certificate or coroner's order had been issued. Also required the registration of stillbirths.
1927	Format of certification changed – new certificates in two parts, the first for the disease or condition leading directly to the cause of death, and causes antecedent to it, and the second for 'other significant conditions contributing to the death, but not related to the disease or condition causing it'.
1931	Adoption of the 4th ICD revision (ICD4).★★
1940	Adoption of the 5th revision of the ICD (ICD5).★★ Major changes made to method of selecting the underlying cause of death when more than one cause was mentioned on the certificate. Now the underlying cause would be selected in accordance with the certifier's preference, as expressed in the order on the certificate.[10]
1950	Adoption of the 6th revision of the ICD.
1958	Adoption of the 7th revision of the ICD.
1968	Adoption of the 8th revision of the ICD.
1978	Criminal Law Act of 1977 – amendments to Rules and Regulations affecting compilation of mortality data for injury and poisoning.[16]
1979	Adoption of the 9th ICD revision.
1981	Registrars work-to-rule (1981–82) significantly affected injury and poisoning data for 1981 and to a lesser extent for 1982, especially cause of injury (no coroners' data).
1984	ONS made a change in their method of applying WHO coding rule 3 – *see* DH2 no 21.[14]
1986	New neonatal death certificate introduced which abandoned the concept of a single underlying cause of death and instead requested separately details of maternal and of fetal contributions to mortality – affects neonatal and all-ages cause-specific mortality data.
1993	Redevelopment of computer systems for processing mortality data, introduction of automatic cause coding. Results: 1) reversal of ONS interpretation of rule 3 (introduced in 1984) to follow internationally agreed rules; 2) medical enquiries suspended until ICD10.
1993	Revised coroner's reporting form introduced in May 1993 – less detail from injury and poisoning deaths.[16]

★OPCS used an unnumbered list instead of the International Classification during 1901–1910.
★★As amended for use in England and Wales.
A listing of the codes and explanations for ICD1–5 used in the ONS Historic Deaths Database is available on CD in text format.
Other factors affecting certification are: improvements in medical diagnosis; improvements in access to care; changes in diagnostic fashion and certification practice.

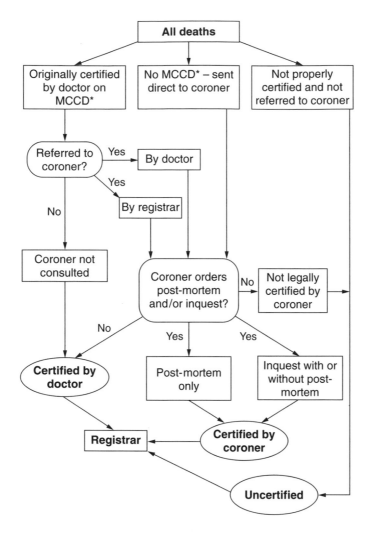

Figure 2.1 Certification and registration of deaths in England and Wales. *Source:* ONS.[3] *Medical certificate of cause of death.

written on the death certificate. These rules are to change markedly in ICD10, and this will have major effects on the number of deaths attributed to many diseases, particularly pneumonias and chronic debilitating diseases such as dementias.

The years for which the ONS has used the various versions are given in Table 2.1. Since the change from the second to third revision there have been 'bridge coding' exercises every time that the classification changed. These exercises have involved coding a sample of death certificates according to both classifications so that the effect of the classification change can be measured, enabling the user to make appropriate adjustments.[8] For example, the user can group together causes in order to get a more consistent series over time.

Problems in identifying the underlying cause of death

Published mortality statistics are usually based on a single, underlying, cause of death, selected by the ONS from the several causes that may be mentioned on the death certificate. Methods for selecting the underlying cause have varied (*see* Table 2.1), and also the number of items on the death certificate has tended to increase, increasing the difficulty in arriving at a single underlying cause.[3] In 1927 the format of death certification changed. The new certificates came in two parts, the first for the disease or condition leading directly to death, and causes antecedent to it, and the second for 'other significant conditions contributing to the death, but not related to the disease or condition causing it'.[7] Figure 2.2 shows the death certificate in current use, much the same as the 1927 certificate. As defined by the ninth revision of the International Classification of Diseases,[7] the underlying cause of death is:

1   the disease or injury that initiated the train of events leading to death, or
2   the circumstances of the accident or violence (e.g. suicide) that produced the fatal injury.

Prior to 1940 the selection of this cause had been determined on the basis of certain rules whereby conditions of various types, for example violence, infectious diseases, and malignant tumours, were given an arbitrary order of precedence, no notice being taken of the order in which the certifying practitioner wrote down the various causes of death.[9] In 1940 the fifth revision of the ICD was adopted, and the ONS made major changes to the method of selecting the underlying cause of death when more than one cause was mentioned on the certificate. Now the underlying cause was to be selected in accordance with the certifier's preference, as expressed in the order on the certificate.[10]

In 1984 ONS made a further change in their method of selecting the underlying cause, using a broader interpretation of the WHO's coding rule 3.[11] This rule states that where the condition in Part I is

19

clearly a direct sequel to a condition in Part II, the latter is to be preferred as the underlying cause. The cause entered in Part II was thus selected more frequently, resulting in a fall in deaths from less specific causes such as bronchopneumonia (ICD 485) and pulmonary embolism (ICD 415.1). The changes resulted in increases in more specific categories, particularly chapters III (Endocrine, nutritional and metabolic and immunity disorders), IV (Blood and blood forming organs), V (Mental disorders), VI (Diseases of the nervous system and sense organs), XII (Diseases of the skin and subcutaneous tissue), and XIII (Diseases of the musculoskeletal system and connective tissue). These changes are discussed in detail elsewhere.[11] In 1993, when automatic cause coding was adopted,[12] the decision taken in 1984 was reversed, moving back to the internationally accepted interpretation operating before 1984. The changes and their effects have been published.[13,14]

Because it can be difficult to select the underlying cause from a multiplicity of recorded causes, the ONS has from time to time produced tables based on more than one cause. The first were in the Registrar General's Annual Reports from 1911 to 1914, the next in the 1931 decennial supplement. The first modern analysis covered a sample of deaths in 1951. Subsequent analyses were published for 1966/67, 1976, and 1985/86, and these have been reintroduced with the availability of automatic cause coded data from 1997 onwards.[15] Here tables include causes *with which* people died as well as those *from which* they died (all causes mentioned on the death certificate). Some conditions such as cancers and cerebrovascular disease frequently appear alone on a death certificate, while causes such as diabetes appear many times more often as 'mentions' than as the underlying cause.[15]

Other considerations affecting interpretation

Problems arise when death certificates do not include sufficient information for accurate cause classification. From 1964 the ONS sent a 'medical inquiry' form to certifying doctors where this occurred, requesting further information. In recent years about 3% of all deaths have been subject to this procedure, with an 80% response rate.[3] Most changes resulting from these were small, and a substantial proportion of these enquiries related to redefinition of the site involved for cancer deaths. Medical enquiries were suspended

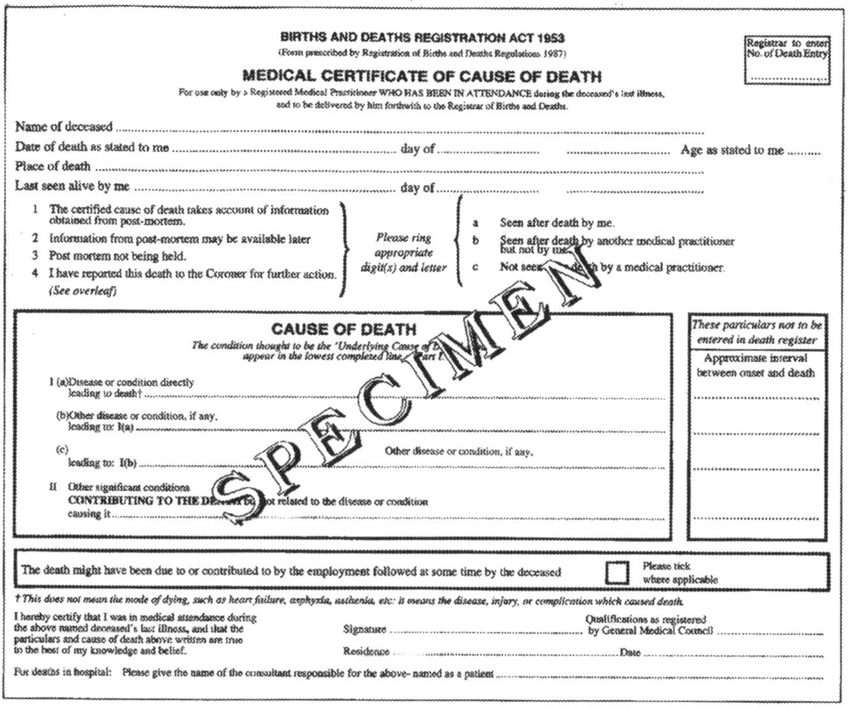

BIRTHS AND DEATHS REGISTRATION ACT 1953
(Form prescribed by Registration of Births and Deaths Regulations 1987)

Registrar to enter No. of Death Entry ....

MEDICAL CERTIFICATE OF CAUSE OF DEATH

For use only by a Registered Medical Practitioner WHO HAS BEEN IN ATTENDANCE during the deceased's last illness, and to be delivered by him forthwith to the Registrar of Births and Deaths.

Name of deceased ....

Date of death as stated to me .... day of .... Age as stated to me ....

Place of death ....

Last seen alive by me .... day of ....

1 The certified cause of death takes account of information obtained from post-mortem.
2 Information from post-mortem may be available later
3 Post mortem not being held.
4 I have reported this death to the Coroner for further action. *(See overleaf)*

Please ring appropriate digit(s) and letter

a Seen after death by me.
b Seen after death by another medical practitioner but not by me.
c Not seen after death by a medical practitioner.

SPECIMEN

CAUSE OF DEATH

The condition thought to be the 'Underlying Cause of Death' should appear in the lowest completed line of Part I.

I (a) Disease or condition directly leading to death† ....

(b) Other disease or condition, if any, leading to: I(a) ....

(c) Other disease or condition, if any, leading to: I(b) ....

II Other significant conditions CONTRIBUTING TO THE DEATH but not related to the disease or condition causing it ....

These particulars not to be entered in death register
Approximate interval between onset and death

The death might have been due to or contributed to by the employment followed at some time by the deceased ☐ Please tick where applicable

† This does not mean the mode of dying, such as heart failure, asphyxia, asthenia, etc: it means the disease, injury, or complication which caused death.

I hereby certify that I was in medical attendance during the above named deceased's last illness, and that the particulars and cause of death above written are true to the best of my knowledge and belief.

Signature .... Qualifications as registered by General Medical Council ....

Residence .... Date ....

For deaths in hospital: Please give the name of the consultant responsible for the above-named as a patient ....

Figure 2.2 Specimen death certificate. *Source*: ONS.

from 1993 but are likely to be reintroduced when ICD10 is implemented.[14]

Data relating to injury and poisoning are particularly complicated. In 1978 the Criminal Law Act of 1977, the Coroners (Amendment) Rules 1977 and the Registration of Births, Deaths and Marriages (Amendment) Regulations altered the rules and regulations affecting compilation of mortality data for deaths from injury and poisoning.[16] The coroner's jury was no longer required to name a person it found guilty of causing a death, and the coroner no longer needed to commit that person for trial. Furthermore, where an inquest is adjourned because a person has been charged with an offence in connection with the death, provisions were made for the death to be registered at the time of adjournment rather than having to wait for the outcome of criminal proceedings. Such deaths were assigned to ICD9 code E988.8 or, in the case of motor vehicle accidents, to the appropriate traffic accident code. The result of this change was that reported homicide deaths were reduced, and open verdicts correspondingly increased – this is discussed in more detail elsewhere.[3]

Furthermore, additional information on causes of death may become available at a later stage, leading to the cause of death being amended. The amended data are used by the ONS in tabulations when available, but amended causes are not shown in the public record, so users with access to individual records of death as shown on the public record (which is not amended) may thus find some differences with published statistics.[16]

Neonatal and fetal deaths

In 1986 new neonatal and fetal death certificates were introduced for stillbirths and deaths occurring in the first 28 days of life. These certificates abandoned the concept of a single underlying cause of death and instead requested separate details of maternal and of fetal contributions to mortality. This affects cause-specific mortality data for deaths of persons under one year of age, since tables by cause now omit deaths in the first 28 days of life. Recently an algorithm has been introduced to derive an underlying cause grouping from the information provided.[17] Scotland has not adopted a new stillbirth and neonatal certificate so this problem in interpreting trends has not arisen there.

Post-mortem examinations

Post-mortem examinations can be a means to a more precise diagnosis. A substantial proportion of death certificates are currently signed without one – 76% in 1992.[3] This figure was 91% in 1928, when statistics on post-mortem examinations first became available. One possible explanation for the decline could be higher levels of diagnostic certainty related to modern investigative techniques prior to death. Post-mortem rates vary according to cause of death, with nearly all coroners' cases (cases of death by injury, poisoning or sudden unexplained death, about a quarter of all deaths) involving post mortems.[3] In 1992 only 2% of doctor-certified deaths that were not referred to the coroner involved post mortems.[3] Deaths from neoplasms, a major cause of death (*see* Chapter 10), rarely require post mortems because diagnoses are usually confirmed by surgery, histology, blood tests and other investigations. Improvements in the accuracy of medical diagnosis, and improvement in access to care may lead to an increase in specific causes (including hard to diagnose conditions such as multiple myeloma), and falls in less specific causes such as symptoms and signs. A large study[18] comparing clinical and autopsy diagnoses of underlying cause of death in the 1960s examined 9501 patients in 75 hospitals in England and Wales and found considerable differences, with agreement in only 45% of cases. However, the overall numbers in most disease groups, regardless of method of diagnosis, were similar, since the errors tended to cancel each other out; for example, 183 patients were coded as dying from malignant diseases on the basis of clinical diagnosis, and 182 by pathologists. A further study some 10 years later of 1126 patients from the Birmingham area comparing autopsy and death certificate diagnoses found 48% complete agreement, 26% partial agreement, and 22% total disagreement.[19]

Alderson[20] has reviewed a number of validation studies to determine the accuracy of cause of death certification for specific diseases, and discussed how these have been affected by changes in diagnosis and coding. There is greater certainty regarding diagnoses in individuals aged under 65, and for men rather than women. In an analysis of data from Bristol, making use of hospital and death certificate data together, he found that in 70% of cases the initial coding was correct, in 20% a minor alteration was required, and in 10% a major alteration. This varied according to whether the certificates were signed by hospital doctors, those recently qualified, those in non-teaching hospitals, and whether the patients were elderly or had respiratory diseases.[21] It was suggested that greater accuracy would result from linking together different data sources such as hospital and mortality data. The Oxford Record Linkage Study[22] is one such linkage exercise.

Population change

Another cause of apparent change in mortality rates, especially crude all-ages rates, is changes that occur in the make-up of the population, for example, when the age distribution changes. If the average age of the population increases then a higher crude mortality is to be expected even if death rates at each single year of age remain constant. This statistical artefact is overcome by 'age standardisation methods', which are necessary to compare mortality levels in different regions or trends across time (*see* Annex 1).

Year of analysis

Up to 1992, deaths recorded in mortality statistics for England and Wales have been those *registered* in England and Wales in calendar periods. From 1993 onwards the ONS has published data by *year of occurrence*. There can be delays in registering a death which vary according to the cause of death, with those involving coroners taking longest. Of the 553 194 deaths that occurred in 1994, less than 2% (or 10 090) were registered after the end of the year. However deaths from injury and poisoning, although accounting for only 2.2% of all deaths, account for 36% of all deaths registered after the end of the calendar year in which they occurred.[23] Generally the effect of this change is small.[14]

Non-residents

No distinction is made between deaths of civilians and non–civilians. The deaths in England and Wales of persons whose usual residence is outside these countries are included in the total figures for England and Wales. Similar procedures apply to Scotland – deaths of English residents in Scotland will appear in Scottish statistics but not English statistics. An assessment of the impact of registration of non-residents on the comparability of mortality statistics, with particular reference to Scotland, has been made.[24] The problems are greater for some causes of deaths (e.g. sudden deaths from heart diseases and accidents) than others (e.g. malignant neoplasms). Deaths of non–residents appear to be more common in Scotland (0.9% of all deaths) than in England and Wales (0.3%). About half of non-resident deaths occur under age 65. Somewhat fewer deaths are referred to the Procurator Fiscal in Scotland than to the coroner in England and Wales, and fewer post mortems are therefore conducted. This may affect the comparability of the data since 'sudden death' is more common in Scotland.[24]

Conclusion

In spite of all the preceding caveats mortality data constitute one of the most important sources of data for monitoring public health, planning, and resource allocation. The data have been universally and regularly collected over a long period of time, and there is no uncertainty about the fact of death. They are one of the only sources available for small geographic areas and the recording is close to being 100% complete. However, in interpreting the statistics it is important to bear in mind the complexity of the recording system, and the potential errors which can be greatly reduced with good training of certifying clinicians.

Acknowledgements

I am grateful to ONS colleagues, especially Tim Devis, for comments on an earlier draft.

References

1   Breeze E, Trevor G and Wilmot A (1991) *General Household Survey 1989*. HMSO, London.
2   Last JM (1963) The iceberg. *Lancet*. **ii**: 28–31.
3   Devis T and Rooney C (1999) Death certification and the epidemiologist. *Health Statistics Quarterly*. **1**: 21–33.
4   ONS (1998) *Mortality Statistics: general 1996*. Series DH1 No. 29. Office for National Statistics, London.
5   Charlton JRH (1986) Use of mortality data in health planning. In: Hansluwka H, Lopez AD and Porapakkham Y *et al.* (eds) *New Developments in the Analysis of Mortality and Causes of Death*. World Health Organization, Mahidol University, Bangkok.
6   Wrigley EA and Schofield RS (1989) *The Population History of England 1541–1871*, 2nd edition. Cambridge University Press, Cambridge.
7   WHO (1977) *Manual of the International Statistical Classification of Diseases, Injuries and Causes of Death, I & II*. World Health Organization, Geneva.
8   OPCS (1983) *Mortality Statistics, comparison of 8th and 9th revisions of the International Classification of Diseases, 1978 (sample) England and Wales*. Series DH1 No. 10. HMSO, London.
9   Logan WPD (1950) Mortality in England and Wales from 1848–1947. *Population Studies*. **4**: 132–78.
10 Campbell H (1965) *Changes in Mortality Trends: England and Wales 1931–1961*. National Center for Health Statistics, Series 3 No. 3. Public Health Service, US DHEW, Washington DC.
11 OPCS (1985) *Mortality Statistics: cause, 1984 England and Wales*. Series DH2 No. 11, p. v–vii. HMSO, London.
12 Birch D (1993) Automatic coding of causes of death. *Population Trends*. **73**: 36–8.
13 Rooney C and Devis T (1996) Mortality trends by cause of death in England and Wales 1980–94: the impact of introducing automated cause coding and related changes in 1993. *Population Trends*. **86**: 29–35.

14   ONS (1996) *Mortality Statistics: cause, 1993 (revised) and 1994.* Series DH2 No. 21. Office for National Statistics, London.

15   ONS (1998) *Mortality Statistics: cause, 1997.* Series DH2 No. 24. Office for National Statistics, London.

16   ONS (1998) *Mortality Statistics: injury and poisoning 1996.* Series DH4 No 21. Office for National Statistics, London.

17   Alberman E, Botting B, Blatchley N *et al.* (1994) A new hierarchical classification of causes of infant death in England and Wales. *Archives of Disease in Childhood.*70: 403–9.

18   Heasman MA and Lipworth L (1966). *Accuracy of Certification of Cause of Death.* OPCS studies in medical and population subjects No. 20. HMSO, London.

19   Waldron HA and Vickerstaff L (1977) *Intimations of Quality: ante mortem and post mortem diagnosis.* Nuffield Provincial Hospitals Trust, London.

20   Alderson MR (1981) *International Mortality Statistics.* Macmillan, London.

21   Alderson MR (1965) The accuracy of certification of death, and the classification of the underlying cause of death from the death certification. London University, MD thesis.

22   Acheson ED (1967) *Medical Record Linkage.* Oxford University Press, Oxford.

23   Devis T and Rooney C (1997) The time taken to register a death. *Population Trends.* 88: 48–55.

24   Carstairs V (1991) Dying away from home: the influence on mortality statistics. *Population Trends.* 66: 22–5.

Annex 1

Definitions of important health indicators calculated by the Office for National Statistics

Age-period cohort analysis

- **Cohort**
  A group of people defined by a selected attribute, often the period in which they were born. This is so that its characteristics can be ascertained as it enters successive time and age periods.

- **Cohort analysis**
  The tabulation and analysis of morbidity and mortality rates in relationship to the birth cohorts of the individuals concerned.

- **Cohort effects (generation effects)**
  Variations in health status that arise from the different causal factors to which each birth cohort in the population is exposed, as the environment and society change. Each cohort is exposed to a different environment that coincides with its life span.

- **Period effects**
  Morbidity and morbidity rates could vary as a result of changes in: the way diseases are recognised and classified by doctors; incidence of disease; efficacy of treatment; coding rules. Such changes are likely to relate to specific periods of time and to affect different generations at the same time. These effects are known as period effects.

- **Age-period cohort analyses**
  These try to disentangle the influences operating over the individual's lifetime from those operating at a specific time on all generations, such as around the date of death. Published mortality tables, for example, give rates by 5-year age groups and year of death, and it is thus possible to calculate the period of birth (year of death minus age at death). Data can thus be plotted against period of death, period of birth or both. There is, however, an identifiability problem in trying to pin down the observed changes to one or the other, since once age of death is known, year of birth and year of death are related by a simple arithmetic formula. If there is a linear decline in mortality it would be impossible to say whether the reason was a period or cohort effect. Various statistical regression based models have been proposed in attempts

to estimate the non-linear effects of period and cohort separately.[1,2] All these models make certain simplifying assumptions in order to produce unique parameter estimates, and these need to be checked for biological plausibility.

Age-specific rate

A rate for a specified age group – the numerator and denominator refer to the same age group. For example, number of deaths among ages 15–24 in a year, divided by the population at risk aged 15–24, multiplied by 1 000 000, gives the death rate per million.

Age-standardised rates and ratios (SMRs)

A procedure for adjusting rates to take account of differences in age composition when comparing rates for different populations, for example, at different dates or between different countries. There are two approaches used: 1. direct standardisation (usually to the standard European population – *see* below); and 2. indirect standardisation, usually expressed as a standardised ratio (for example, standardised mortality ratio). Both methods are based on weighted averaging of rates specific for age, sex, and sometimes other potential confounding variables.

- The *direct method* averages specific rates in a study population using as weights the distribution of a specified population (*see* European population below). This standardised rate represents what the crude rate would have been in the study population if the population had the same distribution as the standard population with respect to the variables for which the adjustment or standardisation was carried out.

  Age-standardised rate $= \sum\sum p_k m_k)/\sum p_k$
  where p_k is the standard population in sex/age group k
  m_k is the observed mortality rate (e.g. deaths per million persons) in sex/age group k
  and k = sex/age group (e.g. 0, 1–4, 5–9,...,85 and over) for males and females.

- The *indirect method* is used to compare study populations for which the specific rates are either statistically unstable or unknown. The specific rates in the standard population are averaged, using as weights the distribution of the study population, to obtain an expected number of events such as deaths. The ratio of the observed events to expected events for the study population is the *standardised mortality* (or *morbidity*) *ratio* or *SMR*. In studying trends, the standard population would typically be one of the years studied, often the first.

SMR = 100 × (observed deaths/expected deaths),
where expected deaths = $\sum p_k m_k$ and
where p_k is the population in sex/age group k in a year
m_k is the mortality rate (deaths per person) in sex/age group k for the standard population/year
and k = sex/age group (e.g. 0, 1–4, 5–9,...,85 and over).

The indirectly standardised rate is the product of the SMR and the crude rate for the standard population.

Another method of adjusting mortality data to take account of the age distribution of a population is the life table – *see* below (for methods *see* Armitage[3]).

Correlation

The degree to which variables change together. A correlation coefficient is a measure of that association, where plus 1 indicates a perfect positive linear relationship and minus 1 represents a perfect negative linear relationship.

Crude death rate

The number of deaths during a specified period, divided by the number at risk during the period. Usually expressed as a rate per million, it provides an estimate of the proportion of the population dying during the specified period (typically per year). It does not take into account the ages of the individuals in the population studied, and can be misleading when examining long-term trends because the age structure of the population may vary over time.

Demographic transition

The transition from high to low fertility (and mortality) rates in a country, formerly thought to be related to technological change (including improved sanitation) and industrialisation but probably more directly related to female literacy and the status of women than to any other factors.[4]

Dependency ratio

The ratio of children and older people in a population to all others, i.e. the proportion of those assumed to be 'economically inactive' to the 'economically active'.

European standard population

This is an artificial population[5] used for direct standardisation of rates. It is in fact reasonably similar to the 1991 England and Wales population (although the age distribution is the same for men and women). The population figures are simplified to make calculations easier.

The standard European population distribution is shown in the table below.

Age group	Standard European Population	Population England & Wales 1991 (Total=100,000)		
		Persons	Males	Females
0	1600	1400	1400	1300
1–4	6400	5300	5600	5100
5–9	7000	6300	6600	6000
10–14	7000	6000	6300	5700
15–19	7000	6400	6700	6100
20–24	7000	7700	8100	7400
25–29	7000	8200	8500	8000
30–34	7000	7300	7500	7100
35–39	7000	6600	6700	6400
40–44	7000	7200	7500	7100
45–49	7000	6200	6400	6000
50–54	7000	5300	5600	5200
55–59	6000	5100	5100	5000
60–64	5000	5000	5000	5100
65–69	4000	4900	4600	5100
70–74	3000	4000	3500	4400
75–79	2000	3300	2600	3900
80–84	1000	2200	1500	2800
85 & over	1000	1600	800	2300
All ages	100 000	100 000	100 000	100 000

Incidence

The rate at which new events occur in the population, i.e. the number of new cases of a disease in a specified period, divided by the population at risk of getting the disease during the period. Often expressed as rates per million population.

International Classification of Diseases

This classification of specific medical conditions and groups of conditions is determined by an internationally representative group of experts who advise the World Health Organization (WHO), which publishes periodic revisions. The ninth revision is currently in use in Britain for mortality, but for some morbidity conditions the tenth (published 1990) is used. Every disease is assigned a code number, and in the ninth revision these are grouped into 17 chapters. In addition there is a classification of injury and poisoning by the external causes of injury, for example, type of accident or suicide.

Life table

A summarising technique used to describe the pattern of mortality and survival in populations. It describes: 1. out of an initial population of 100 000 live births, how many persons survive to age x (l_x); 2. the average number of further years of life remaining to persons who survive to age x (e^0_x); and 3. the proportion alive at age x who die between age x and $x+1$ years (nq_x). Life expectation at birth is often used as a general health status measure for a population. One advantage of this measure is that it is readily understood by the general public. The survival data relate to a specific time, and it is assumed that the individuals in the table are subject throughout life to the age-specific death rates in question. Two types of life table exist.

- Current or period life tables are a summary of mortality experience over a brief period (one to three years), and the population data relate to the middle of that period. It represents the combined mortality experience by age of the population over the short period.

- Cohort or generation life tables describe the actual survival experience of a group, or cohort, of individuals born at about the same time. Theoretically, the mortality experiences of the persons in the cohort would be observed from their moment of birth through each consecutive age in successive calendar years until all of them die. In practice actuarial techniques are used to project future mortality based on changing patterns in the past. Life tables are also classified according to the length of age interval in which the data are presented. A complete life table contains data for every single year of age from birth. An abridged life table contains data by intervals of 5 or 10 years of age. It should be noted that survival is cumulative; for example, the value of l_{40}, survivorship by age 40, is determined by the cumulative age-specific death rates for all ages below 40.

A basic assumption that is made in constructing the life table is that the death rates used are applicable throughout the period. If there is significant in- or out-migration of healthy or unhealthy individuals this could affect the interpretation of the life table. Life tables for England and Wales are described in detail by Devis.[6]

Odds ratio

The ratio of two odds, usually used when comparing risks among cases and controls. It measures the ratio of the odds in favour of exposure among the cases to the odds in favour of exposure among the controls.

Potential years of life lost (PYLL)

This is a measure of the relative impact of various diseases on premature mortality. PYLL highlights the loss to society as a result of early deaths (e.g. below age 65 or 75). The figure is the sum, over all persons dying from that cause, of the years that those persons would have lived had they survived to the stated age (e.g. 65).

Prevalence rate

This is the number of people with a disease at a given time (point prevalence) or at any time in a specified period (period prevalence), divided by the number of people at risk from that disease. Often expressed as rates per million. Lifetime prevalence is another form of period prevalence.

Proportional mortality ratio (PMR)

This is the proportion of observed deaths from a specified condition in a defined population (e.g. an occupation), divided by the proportion of deaths expected from that condition in a standard population with that age/sex composition. The calculation is essentially the same as that for standardised mortality ratios (SMRs), but the number of deaths from all causes replaces the population figures in the calculations. Thus the m_ks in the SMR formula become the proportion of all deaths in the reference population that are due to a specified condition in the PMR formula, and the number of deaths from all causes in the study population become the p_ks. Note that in any segment of the population a high PMR is compatible with a low underlying death rate.

Regression analysis

Given data on a dependent variable y and one or more independent variables x_1, x_2,...,x_x regression analysis involves fitting the 'best' mathematical model (within some restricted class of models) to predict y from the xs. Most common in epidemiology are ordinary linear models, logistic, Poisson, and proportional hazards models.

Sex ratio

The ratio of male to female rates, usually expressed as a percentage. For example, if the mortality sex ratio for a particular age range is 200 then males are twice as likely to die in that age range as females.

References

1   Clayton DG and Schifflers E (1987) Models for temporal variation in cancer rates I: age-period and age-cohort models. *Statistics in Medicine*. 6: 449–67.

2   Lee WC and Lin RS (1995) Analysis of cancer rates using excess risk age-period-cohort models. *International Journal of Epidemiology*. 24(4): 671–7.

3   Armitage P (1971) *Statistical Methods in Medical Research*. Blackwell, New York.

4   Last JM (1995) *A Dictionary of Epidemiology*, 3rd edition. Oxford University Press, Oxford.

5   World Health Organization (1991) World Health Annual Statistics – based on J Waterhouse *et al.* (eds) (1976) *Cancer Incidence in Five Continents*. International Agency for Research on Cancer, Lyons. WHO, Geneva.

6   Devis T (1990) The expectation of life in England and Wales. *Population Trends*. 60: 23–4.

3   ONS data: other health sources

John Charlton

Chapter 2 covered statistics on death, the ultimate level of adverse health, but health monitoring also requires measures of incidence, prevalence, severity of illnesses, and the consequences of illness, classified by age, sex, socio–economic and geographical character-istics of the population. There are no ideal measures, and several sources are used in combination. The varied sources of population health information provide different pieces of the overall health jigsaw. The Office for National Statistics (ONS) publishes decennial reviews from time to time that combine data from all sources to provide a more complete picture of health, for example *The Health of Adult Britain*,[1] and *The Health of our Children*.[2] Up to date information on UK government publications and data can be found on STATBASE (http://www.statistics.gov.uk).

Censuses and population estimates

It is difficult to interpret counts of medical events without adequate population denominators against which rates can be calculated. The first national census of population was conducted in 1801, with further censuses at 10-year intervals apart from 1941. There was, however, population registration in 1939. The 1841 Census was the first to be conducted by the Registrar General, when the method of enumeration changed from a count of houses and persons by local Overseers of the Poor to self-enumeration by household, directed by the registration service. As well as counts of the population by age and sex, the census has provided a wealth of information about the socio–economic characteristics of the population such as household composition, marital status, education, employment, accommoda-tion and lack of amenities, enabling trends to be studied. Some health questions have been asked from time to time: from 1851 to 1911 the number of 'idiots', blind, deaf and dumb were enumerated, and in 1991 a question was included on limiting long-term illness (LLTI). The availability and validity of past census data have been reviewed.[3] Since 1961 it has been standard practice for the ONS to carry out a census evaluation programme, to check the coverage and quality of replies entered on the census form. The method used is to repeat the enumeration for a sample of the households shortly after census day, using a team of skilled interviewers. In 1981 the net under-enumeration was 0.5%. In 1991 there was an estimated 1% shortfall, which was concentrated in men and to a lesser extent women aged from 19 to 30.[4] The discrepancy was as high as 6% at age 27, and it is thought that avoidance of the recently introduced and unpopular 'poll tax' was a factor.

Between census years annual mid-year estimates are produced which take account of births, deaths, and migration into and out of the country, local and health authorities.[5] The methodology includes using data from the International Passenger Survey for international migration, the National Health Service Central Register for movements between Family Health Services Authorities, electoral roll statistics, and comparison of censuses for the Republic of Ireland and Great Britain. Population projections for future years are also made.[6,7] ONS, previously OPCS (Office of Population Censuses and Surveys), continually monitors the accuracy of its estimates.[8]

The population covered by population estimates has varied over time. From 1915 to 1920 and from 3 September 1939 to 31 December 1949 for men and 1 June 1941 to 31 December 1949 for women only the civilian population was covered – excluding all members of HM Forces and Forces of other countries stationed in England and Wales. Between 1950 and 1970 the population estimates related to the home population – those living in England and Wales, including overseas visitors to the country and the Forces of other countries temporarily in England and Wales, but excluding residents and members of HM Forces who were outside the country on census night. From 1971 onwards the estimates relate to the resident population – those resident in England and Wales including members of HM and non-UK Forces stationed in England and Wales, and residents who were outside the country on census night, but excluding overseas visitors and HM and non-UK Forces stationed outside the country.

Notifications of infectious diseases

National notification of infectious diseases was introduced with the Infectious Diseases Notification Act of 1889, which aimed to combat 'dangerous infectious disorders'. In Scotland notification was introduced two years earlier.[9] These data are now collected by the Communicable Disease Surveillance Centre for England and Wales, and the Scottish Centre for Infection and Environmental Health in Scotland. Data on other infectious diseases not notifiable under statute are collected through voluntary laboratory reporting by microbiologists (e.g. salmonella infections, influenza and HIV) and voluntary confidential clinical reporting systems (e.g. for AIDS). Details of cases reported by laboratories include age, sex, diagnosis, time and place of diagnosis. AIDS case reports include data on risk factors for HIV infection and clinical status of the patient at the time of diagnosis.[10] Notification of infectious diseases is recognised as being far from complete, especially for those conditions considered to be less severe or of lesser public health importance.[11] Studies have shown that tuberculosis notifications were accurate to within 10%,[12] for measles some 40–60% of cases were reported,[13] whereas for pertussis only between 5 and 25% were. Significant under-reporting has also been found with notifications of meningitis.[14] Influenza was under-reported as the underlying cause of death until there was an epidemic, when it tended to become over-reported.[15] In England and Wales the Royal College of General Practitioners collects data on patients with infectious diseases via a group of 'spotter' general practices who report on cases encountered.[16,17] A similar scheme operates in Scotland.

Cancer registrations: role of the ONS

The national system of cancer registration is largely covered in Chapter 10. There is a two-way flow of information between the ONS and the regional registries. This enhances the performance, and extends the contribution, of both systems.

The majority of cases for which the registries hold information are derived from hospital sources of data. This is supplemented by information from the ONS, which provides the registries with copies of any death drafts (Form 310) that mention cancer. In return a standard dataset is submitted by the registries to the ONS.

The ONS is also responsible for: flagging, at the NHS Central Register, cases submitted by registries; providing regional registries with death drafts of flagged cases dying from causes other than cancer; and the editing, processing, analysis and publication of national statistics on cancer registration and survival. For England and Wales this has been described in detail elsewhere.[18,19] In Scotland a similar system is coordinated by the Information Services Division of the Scottish Health Service Common Services Agency.

Prior to 1971, registration data were published in the Registrar General's Statistical Review of England and Wales, Supplements on Cancer. Since 1971 registration data have been linked with information on deaths in the NHS Central Register. This permits automatic identification of the fact of death, thereby facilitating calculation of survival statistics, and relieving the cancer registries of the need for ad-hoc follow-up through hospitals and general practitioners.

Since 1971, cancer registration statistics have been published annually by the OPCS, and later the ONS, in the MB1 series of reports. The 1994 publication includes trends for 1979 to 1989 and a commentary on the major cancer sites,[18] and a monitor series on survival is available. Trends for earlier time periods are presented in the ONS publication on cancer registration surveillance 1968 to 1978,[19] and by the Cancer Research Campaign's report for Great Britain.[20] Data for Scotland are published by the Scottish NHS.[21,22]

Congenital anomalies

Partly as a result of the thalidomide epidemic of 1960 a national notification scheme was started in England and Wales in 1964, whereby doctors and midwives notified the local medical officer of health about any congenital anomaly identifiable at birth or within 7 days, later extended to 10 days. This time limit has recently been removed. These data are forwarded to ONS for analysis.[23,24] The validity of these data has been reviewed.[3,25] Although there is under-notification and evidence of potential biases in notification, this varies according to the malformation; the most easily recognised ones have the most complete recording. The data were judged to be of sufficient quality to expose any increase in incidence.

Abortions

Abortion data when combined with data on births can provide information on teenage pregnancies and other important health issues relating to women and their babies, for example, on the occurrence of neural tube defects.[26] Statistics on 'conceptions' are produced combining abortion data with data on live and stillbirths, based on the estimated year of conception. Reducing the number of conceptions to mothers under age 16 is a *Health of the Nation* target. Similar data are processed for Scotland by the Information and Statistics Division. The concern about rising maternal mortality in the 1930s drew attention to the consequences of illegal abortion since at that time between 16 and 20% of pregnancies ended in abortion.[27] The 1967 Abortion Act came into operation in Britain in April 1968, and requires notifications of termination of pregnancy to be made to the Chief Medical Officers within 7 days. ONS processes these data on behalf of the Department of Health. Limited abortion data were available, from 1949, from the Hospital In-Patient Enquiry (HIPE). Information is available on the woman's age, marital status, place of residence, number of previous children, length of gestation, statutory grounds for termination, and methods used. Botting[28] has reviewed the trends since 1968. The rapid increase between 1968 and 1972 is likely to be largely due to transfer of abortions from the illegal to the legal sector, and changing patterns of abortions to non-residents of England and Wales. In more recent years, however, the increase may have been influenced, at least in part, by changing fertility patterns, the changing age structure of the population of fertile women, changing contraception patterns, and changing attitudes towards abortion. Birth and maternity statistics are discussed in Chapter 9.

General practice records

There is a vast amount of health-related data available from GP and hospital records (*see* Chapter 4 for a discussion of hospital activity data). The ONS has jointly undertaken National Morbidity Studies in General Practice in conjunction with the Royal College of General Practitioners at 10-year intervals.[29] The General Practice Research Database,[30,31] owned by the Secretary of State for Health and managed by the Medicines Control Agency, continuously collects data from about 400 practices in the UK, and is the largest dataset of its kind in the world. Primary care data in general are discussed in Chapter 5.

The general practitioner is gate-keeper to health services (except for emergencies and genitourinary medicine), and thus utilisation data collected from this source should give us the most comprehensive picture of overall health service utilisation. However, in deciding whether to consult a general practitioner, a patient may be influenced by a number of factors: their perception of the severity of the problem; the expectation that they might be helped; the accessibility of the surgery premises; the need for sickness certification; and the availability of alternative sources of care such as accident and emergency departments and family planning clinics. The data thus measure individuals' expressed need for GP care. They can also be heavily influenced by organisational changes; for example, a shift of routine care from hospitals to GP care, as has happened with diabetic care, could result in an artefactual increase in prevalence of the disease treated, according to the GP data, but a reduction according to the hospital data.

The first national GP-based morbidity survey was conducted by Logan and Cushion in 1955/56.[32] The second and third studies were conducted in 1970/76.[33–37] The two most recent morbidity surveys, in 1981 and 1991/92, surveyed 300 000 and 500 000 persons respectively. Until 1991 the studies required GPs to record morbidity in the form of special manual records. The 1991/92 survey, however, recruited practices that routinely recorded all their consultation data on computers.[29] The survey covered 1% of the population of England and Wales. The patients were similar in terms of age and socio-economic characteristics to the population of England and Wales, as recorded in the 1991 Census, although the practices tended to have larger lists and younger GPs than the average. The Weekly Returns Service (WRS) of the Royal College of General Practitioners monitors the incidence of new disease presented to general practitioners each week.[38] Ninety two practices with a combined population of approximately 700 000 persons record new episodes of illness and report the numbers in age and sex groups on each Wednesday for the previous week. The data are aggregated at the General Practice Research Unit in Birmingham. The practices are well distributed nationally and data are presented in three supra-regional groups – North, Central and South. There are currently a number of other databases collecting data from general practices on a continuous basis, one of the most important being the General Practice Research Database (GPRD), which the Medicines Control Agency (MCA) manages. In addition, health authorities are working with GPs in their areas to collect data in order to assess local needs. GP morbidity data from national samples have also been used in conjunction with census data to produce estimates of local morbidity.[39]

Although the quality of GP data is sometimes criticised, internal consistency has been illustrated in regional analysis of data for allergic rhinitis for 1992, a year in which incidence rates of allergic rhinitis were particularly high.[40] Comparability with specialist diagnosis is demonstrated in an examination of data for hospital discharges with a diagnosis of asthma and new episodes presenting to general practitioners.[41] Laboratory validation of GP diagnoses is illustrated by comparing the incidence of influenzal illness with the results of virological investigation.[42] Although there may be a time lag for laboratory reports, it is valuable to use such different sources in conjunction to confirm validity. The GPRD data have also been validated and found to be of good quality.[30] This is discussed further in Chapter 5.

Linked routinely collected data

The ONS Longitudinal Study[43] is based on a 1% sample of the usually resident population of England and Wales, and commenced with a sample taken from the 1971 decennial census. This consists of all individuals born on four specific days in the year. Data are linked to this sample from different routine sources. The study relies to a large extent on tracing individuals through the National Health Service Central Register (NHSCR). New births occurring on the four days in the year, and immigrants who register with the NHS who were born on these days, are added to the sample so that it continues to represent 1% of the population. For each individual the following events are linked: live and stillbirths to women in the sample; deaths under one year of age of these children; immigration and emigration; death of a spouse; cancer registrations; death; and census data from subsequent years. The main value of this study is that it is possible to analyse changes over time using data on individuals, and it is relatively easy to perform exploratory analyses quickly in response to specific questions that arise from time to time, free from numerator/denominator biases. It has made significant contributions in the field of occupational mortality,[43] because the occupation of women is not always recorded on the death certificate, and men and women change occupations over time. It is particularly valuable in analysing socio-economic data in relation to mortality.

As has already been mentioned, since the 1970s all cancer notifications have been sent to the NHSCR and subsequently linked to death records.[44,45] Another use that has been made of the NHSCR has been to link data on various kinds of exposure to subsequent mortality, for example in occupational mortality studies.[46] An early example of this was when a relationship was found between exposure to dyestuff of workers in the chemical industry and bladder tumours.[47] The Oxford Record Linkage Study[48] links hospitalisation records of individuals together, and to birth, death and cancer registration records. The Scottish Record Linkage System is somewhat different.[49]

Survey data

Surveys provide subjective information on health from the point of view of individuals in the population, as well as more objective information if physical examination is combined with the interview. They are important in filling in gaps in knowledge about health status, behaviour and attitudes that the routine sources cannot satisfy. Provided the sample is well designed they provide detailed information on individuals that is representative of the population surveyed. A number of surveys are discussed below – the datasets are deposited in the ESRC Data Archive (*see* Chapter 6). The Health Survey for England is discussed in Chapter 7.

General Household Survey (GHS)

The GHS is a valuable ongoing annual household survey of some 17 000 individuals that has been conducted by the ONS since 1971.[50] It includes some core questions on general health, long-standing illnesses and whether these limit the respondent's activities, and socio-economic characteristics. Questions on health-related behaviours such as smoking and drinking are included every other year, as well as additional health-related questions from time to time. The survey is one of the main means of tracking trends in smoking and drinking behaviours, perceptions of general health, utilisation of health services in relation to individual socio-economic characteristics, ethnic group, etc. From time to time there is a supplement on topics such as activities of daily living among the elderly.

The ONS Omnibus Survey

The Omnibus Survey is a monthly survey, sampling some 2000 individuals aged 16 and over in private households every month. Different organisations commission questions which run for however many months they are required. For example, in 1995 the Department of Health commissioned questions on general health, including the EuroQol (a quality of life measure). The survey is particularly useful for establishing people's attitudes, and the results are made available shortly after the survey.

The ONS Disability Surveys

The Disability Surveys, the most recent of which was carried out in 1985–88, give information on the type and severity of disabling conditions, by age and sex.[51] They cover private households and communal establishments, but do not provide information on the prevalence of the conditions causing the disability. They have provided important information for the formulation of health policy.

The Labour Force Survey (LFS)

The LFS has been carried out in the UK since 1973.[52] Up to 1983 it was biennial, from 1984 to 1991 it was annual, and from 1992 it has been carried out quarterly, and is the largest survey conducted by the ONS. It covers all persons normally resident in private households in the UK, and each individual is included for five successive quarters. It includes a wealth of socio-economic information, ethnic group, education, employment, and some measures of health such as limiting longstanding illness, sickness absence, and health problems that affect work.

The ONS Psychiatric Morbidity Surveys

The Psychiatric Morbidity Surveys were commissioned by the Department of Health, the Scottish Office and the Health Department of the Welsh Office to provide information about the prevalence of psychiatric problems in the population, as well as their associated social disabilities and use of services. Carried out between 1993 and 1995, they provide a measure of prevalence of minor and severe mental health problems in the general population, as well as the population in institutions and the homeless.[53-57] Analyses by socio-economic characteristics were undertaken which showed wide variations, with more socially disadvantaged persons bearing greater burdens.

Health in England[58]

Health in England Surveys of adults aged between 16 and 74 are carried out by the ONS on behalf of the Health Education Authority. The aim is to monitor what people know, think and do in relation to healthy lifestyles, in order to measure progress towards *Health of the Nation* targets. Also included are questions on self-reported general health, whether they led a healthy life, stress, and self-reported morbidity.

Dental Health Surveys[59-68]

Dental Health Surveys were conducted by the ONS in 1968, 1978 and 1988. They showed, for example, that in 1968 29% of all adults had no natural teeth, with worse dental health in the North than the South, but by 1978 dental health had much improved – to different extents in different parts of the country.

Food Surveys

Food Surveys have collected data from the middle of the nineteenth century, initially to monitor the nutrition of the less well-off, but the early data sources may not be strictly comparable with later surveys, and were often based on small samples. Larger more recent surveys carried out by the ONS were: The Dietary and Nutritional Survey of British Adults;[69] The National Diet and Nutrition Survey of Children aged 1½ to 4½ years.[70]

Some other surveys by the ONS relating to health

There are many other surveys that are of relevance to health, but space does not permit describing them all. They include:

- heights and weights of British adults[71]
- people aged 65 and over[72]
- smoking among secondary school children in England[73-80]

- drinking in Britain[81–84]
- survey of the physical health of prisoners.[85]

Syntheses of survey and other health data

The ONS has combined data from several sources, for example to examine health expectancy – disability-free life expectancy.[86] This combines data from the GHS and disability surveys with life tables to produce tables giving estimates of life expectation without disability. Other syntheses of datasets have been produced; for example, data from the Morbidity Statistics from the General Practice Survey have been combined with data from the Census Sample of Anonymised Records to produce local estimates.[87]

References

1   Charlton JRH and Murphy M (1997) *The Health of Adult Britain 1841–1994. Volumes 1 and 2.* ONS, London.
2   Botting B (1995) *The Health of our Children.* ONS, London.
3   Ashley JSA, Cole SK and Kilbane MPJ (1991) Health information resources: United Kingdom – health and social factors. In: *Oxford Textbook of Public Health Volume II.* pp. 29–53. Oxford University Press, Oxford.
4   OPCS (1993) How complete was the 1991 Census? *Population Trends.* **71**: 22–5.
5   OPCS (1993) Rebasing the annual population estimates. *Population Trends.* **73**: 27–31.
6   Daykin C (1986) Projecting the population of the United Kingdom. *Population Trends.* **44**: 28.
7   Armitage RI (1986) Population projections for English local authority areas. *Population Trends.* **43**: 31.
8   OPCS (1982) *A Comparison of the Registrar General's Annual Population Estimates for England and Wales Compared with the Results of the 1981 Census.* Occasional Paper No. 29. Office of Population Censuses and Surveys, London.
9   McCormick A (1993) The notification of infectious diseases in England and Wales. *CDR Review.* 3(2): R19–25.
10 McCormick A, Tillett H, Bannister B *et al.* (1987) Surveillance of AIDS in the United Kingdom. *British Medical Journal.* 295:1466–9.
11 Haward RA (1973) Scale of under notification of infectious diseases by general practitioners. *Lancet.* i(7808): 873–8.
12 Davies PDO, Darbyshire J, Nunn AJ *et al.* (1981) Ambiguities and

inaccuracies in the notification system for tuberculosis in England and Wales. *Community Medicine.* **3:** 108–18.

13 Clarkson JA and Fine PFM (1985) The efficiency of measles and pertussis morbidity reporting in England and Wales. *International Journal of Epidemiology.* **14:** 153–68.

14 Goldacre MJ and Miller DL (1976) Completeness of statutory notification of acute bacterial meningitis. *British Medical Journal.* 2(6034): 501–3.

15 Tillett E and Spencer IL (1982) Influenza surveillance in England and Wales using routine statistics. *Journal of Hygiene.* **88:** 33.

16 Fleming DM (1991) Measurement of morbidity in general practice. *Journal of Epidemiology and Community Health.* **45:** 180–3.

17 Fleming DM, Crombie DL and Ross AM (1996) *Weekly Returns Service Report for 1995.* Birmingham Research Unit of the Royal College of General Practitioners, Birmingham.

18 OPCS (1994) *Cancer Statistics: registrations 1989.* Series MB1 No. 22. HMSO, London.

19 OPCS (1983) *Cancer Registration Surveillance 1968–78 England and Wales.* HMSO, London.

20 CRC (1982) *Trends in Cancer Survival in Great Britain: cases registered between 1960 and 1974.* Cancer Research Campaign, London.

21 Black R, Sharp L and Kendrick SW (1993) *Trends in Cancer Survival in Scotland 1968–90.* Information and Statistics Division, Directorate of Information Services. National Health Service in Scotland, Edinburgh.

22 Sharp L, Black RJ, Harkness EF *et al.* (1993) *Cancer Registration Statistics Scotland 1981–1990.* Scottish Cancer Intelligence Unit, Information and Statistics Division, Directorate of Information Services. National Health Service in Scotland, Edinburgh.

23 Weatherall JAC (1978) Congenital malformations: surveillance and reporting. *Population Trends.* **11:** 27.

24 Botting B (1995) Congenital anomalies. In: Botting B (ed) *The Health of our Children,* Decennial Supplement, Series DS No. 11. HMSO, London.

25 Morris J, Mutton DE, Ide R *et al.* (1994) Monitoring trends in prenatal diagnosis of Down's syndrome in England and Wales, 1989–92. *Journal of Medical Screening.* **1:** 233–7.

26 Hey K, O'Donnell M, Murphy M *et al.* (1994) Use of local neural tube defect registers to interpret national trends. *Archives of Disease in Childhood.* **71:** 198–202.

27 Report of Committee on Medical Aspects of Abortion (1936) *British Medical Journal.* **1**(Suppl.): 230–8.

28 Botting B (1991) Trends in abortion. *Population Trends.* **64:** 19–29.

29 McCormick A, Fleming D and Charlton J (1995) *Morbidity Statistics from General Practice: fourth national study 1991–92*. Series MB5 No. 3. HMSO, London.

30 Hollowell J (1997) The General Practice Research Database: quality of morbidity data. *Population Trends*. 87: 36–40.

31 ONS (1998) *Key Health Statistics from General Practice*. ONS, London.

32 General Register Office (1958) *Morbidity Statistics from General Practice, 1955–6 (vols I–III)*. Studies on Medical and Population Subjects No. 14. HMSO, London.

33 RCGP, OPCS and DoH (1974) *Morbidity Statistics from General Practice: second national study, 1970–71*. Studies on Medical and Population Subjects No. 26. HMSO, London.

34 RCGP, OPCS and DoH (1979) *Morbidity Statistics from General Practice, 1971–72: Second national study*. Studies on Medical and Population Subjects No. 36. HMSO, London.

35 RCGP, OPCS and DoH (1982) *Morbidity Statistics from General Practice, 1970–71: socio-economic analysis*. Studies on Medical and Population Subjects No. 46. HMSO, London.

36 RCGP, OPCS and DoH (1986) *Morbidity Statistics from General Practice: third national study, 1981–82*. Series MB5 no. 1. HMSO, London.

37 RCGP, OPCS and DoH (1990). *Morbidity Statistics from General Practice. Third morbidity study: socioeconomic analysis 1981–82*. Series MB5 No. 2. HMSO, London.

38 Fleming DM, Norbury CA and Crombie DL (1991) *Annual and Seasonal Variation in the Incidence of Common Diseases*. Occasional Paper 53. Royal College of General Practitioners, London.

39 Charlton JRH, Heady P and Nicolaas G (1995) Demand for General Practitioner Services – a practical test of synthesised estimation. In: *Data Needs in an Era of Health Reform, Proceedings of the 25th Public Health Conference on Records and Statistics 1995*. US Department of Health and Human Services, Washington DC.

40 Ross AM and Fleming DM (1994) Incidence of allergic rhinitis in general practice, 1981–92. *British Medical Journal*. 308: 897–900.

41 LAIA (1993) *Seasonal Variations in Asthma*. Factsheet 93/4. Lung and Asthma Information Agency, Department of Public Health Sciences, St George's Hospital Medical School, Cranmer Terrace, London SW17 0RE.

42 Fleming DM (1996) The impact of three influenza epidemics on primary care in England and Wales. *PharmacoEconomics*. 9(Suppl. 3): 38–45.

43 Fox AJ and Goldbladtt PO (1982) *Socio-demographic Differentials in Mortality*. Longitudinal study series, LS No. 1. HMSO, London.

44   OPCS (1970) *Report of the Advisory Committee on Cancer Registration.* Office of Population Censuses and Surveys, London.

45   OPCS (1981) *Report of the Advisory Committee on Cancer Registration.* Series MB1 No. 6. HMSO, London.

46   OPCS (1993) *Uses of OPCS Records for Medical Research.* OPCS Occasional Paper 41. Office of Population Censuses and Surveys, London.

47   Case RAM and Pearson JT (1954) Tumours of the urinary bladder in workmen engaged in the manufacture and use of certain dyestuff intermediates in the British Chemical Industry. *British Journal of Industrial Medicine.* **11**: 213–32.

48   Acheson ED (1967) *Medical Record Linkage.* Oxford University Press, Oxford.

49   Kendrick S and Clarke J (1993) The Scottish record linkage system. *Health Bulletin.* **51**(2): 72–9.

50   OPCS (1995) *Living in Britain. Preliminary results from the 1994 General Household Survey.* HMSO, London.

51   Martin J, Meltzer H and Elliot D (1988) *The Prevalence of Disability Among Adults: OPCS surveys of disability in Great Britain (Report 1).* HMSO, London.

52   OPCS (1992) *Labour Force Survey 1990 and 1991.* HMSO, London.

53   Meltzer H, Gill B, Petticrew M *et al.* (1995) *OPCS Surveys of Psychiatric Morbidity in Great Britain, Report 1. The prevalence of psychiatric morbidity among adults living in private households.* HMSO, London.

54   Meltzer H, Gill B, Petticrew M *et al.* (1995) *OPCS Surveys of Psychiatric Morbidity in Great Britain, Report 2. Physical complaints, service use and treatment of adults with psychiatric disorders.* HMSO, London.

55   Meltzer H *et al.* (1996) *The Prevalence of Psychiatric Morbidity Among Adults Living in Institutions.* ONS, London.

56   Gill B *et al.* (1996) *Psychiatric Morbidity Among Homeless People.* ONS, London.

57   Meltzer H *et al.* (1998). *Psychiatric Morbidity Among Prisoners in England and Wales.* ONS, London.

58   Bridgwood A, Malbon G, Lader D *et al.* (1996) *Health in England 1995.* HMSO, London.

59   Todd JE and Whitworth A (1974) *Adult Dental Health in Scotland 1972.* Social Survey Report SS1009. HMSO, London.

60   Todd JE (1975) *Children's Dental Health in England and Wales 1973.* Social Survey Report SS1011. HMSO, London.

61   Todd JE and Walker AM (1980) *Adult Dental Health Vol 1: England and Wales, 1968–78.* Social Survey Report SS1112. HMSO, London.

62   Todd JE, Walker AM and Dodd T (1982) *Adult Dental Health. Vol. 2: United Kingdom 1978.* Social Survey Report SS1112. HMSO, London.

63 Todd JE and Dodd T (1985) *Children's Dental Health in the United Kingdom 1983.* Social Survey Report SS1189 HMSO, London.

64 Todd JE (1988) *Scottish Children's Dental Health 1983–1986.* Social Survey Report SS1211. HMSO, London.

65 Todd JE and Lader D (1991) *Adult Dental Health 1988: United Kingdom.* Social Survey Report SS1260. HMSO, London.

66 Todd J, Lader D and Dodd T (1994) *Dental Crowns: report of a follow-up to the 1988 Adult Dental Health Survey.* HMSO, London.

67 O'Brien M (1994) *Children's Dental Health in the United Kingdom 1993.* Social Survey Report SS1350. HMSO, London.

68 Hinds K and Gregory JR (1995) *National Diet and Nutrition Survey: children aged 1½ to 4½ years: volume 2: report of the dental survey.* HMSO, London.

69 Gregory J, Foster K, Tyler H *et al.* (1990) *The Dietary and Nutritional Survey of British Adults.* HMSO, London.

70 Gregory J, Collins D, Davies P *et al.* (1995) *National Diet and Nutritional Survey: children aged 1½ to 4½ years.* HMSO, London.

71 Knight I (1984) *The Heights and Weights of Adults in Great Britain.* HMSO, London.

72 Goddard E and Savage D (1994) *People Aged 65 and Over: a study carried out on behalf of the Department of Health as part of the 1991 General Household Survey* (Series GHS No. 22; suppl A). HMSO, London.

73 Dobbs J and Marsh A (1983) *Smoking Among Secondary School Children: an enquiry carried out for the Department of Health and Social Security, the Welsh Office and the Scottish Home and Health Department.* HMSO, London.

74 Dobbs J and Marsh A (1985) *Smoking Among Secondary School Children in 1984: an enquiry carried out for the Department of Health and Social Security, the Welsh Office and the Scottish Home and Health Department.* HMSO, London.

75 Goddard E and Ikin C (1987) *Smoking Among Secondary School Children in 1986: an enquiry carried out by the Social Survey Division of OPCS on behalf of the Department of Social Security, the Welsh Office and the Scottish Home and Health Department.* HMSO, London.

76 Goddard E (1989) *Smoking Among Secondary School Children in 1988: an enquiry carried out by the Social Survey Division of OPCS on behalf of the Department of Health.* HMSO, London.

77 Bolling K (1994) *Smoking Among Secondary School Children in 1993: an enquiry carried out by the Social Survey Division of OPCS on behalf of the Department of Health.* HMSO, London.

78 Diamond A and Goddard E (1995) *Smoking Among Secondary School Children in 1994: an enquiry carried out by the Social Survey Division of*

OPCS on behalf of the Department of Health, the Welsh Office and the Scottish Home and Health Department. HMSO, London.

79   Lader D and Matheson J (1991) *Smoking Amongst Secondary School Children in 1990.* HMSO, London.

80   Thomas M, Holroyd S and Goddard E (1993) *Smoking Among Secondary School Children in 1992.* HMSO, London.

81   Wilson P (1980) *Drinking in England and Wales: an enquiry carried out on behalf of the Department of Health and Social Security.* OPCS, London.

82   Goddard E (1991) *Drinking in England and Wales in the Late 1980s: an enquiry carried out by Social Survey Division of OPCS on behalf of the Department of Health in association with the Home Office.* HMSO, London.

83   Dight SE (1976) *Scottish Drinking Habits and Attitudes Towards Alcohol, carried out in 1972 for the Scottish Home and Health Department.* HMSO, London.

84   Marsh A, Dobbs J and White A (1986) *Adolescent Drinking: a survey carried out on behalf of the Department of Health and Social Security and the Scottish Home and Health Department.* HMSO, London.

85   Bridgwood A and Malbon G (1995) *Survey of the Physical Health of Prisoners 1994: a survey of sentenced male prisoners in England and Wales, carried out by the Social Survey Division of OPCS on behalf of the Prison Service Health Care Directorate.* Social Survey Report 1376. OPCS, London

86   Bone MR, Bebbington AC, Jagger C *et al.* (1995) *Health Expectancy and its Uses.* HMSO, London.

87   Charlton J and Heady P (1995) Estimating local needs for GP services – a practical test of synthesised estimates. In: *Data Needs in an Era of Health Reform, Proceedings of the 25th Public Health Conference on Records and Statistics 1995.* US Department of Health and Human Services, Washington DC.

4 Hospital Episode Statistics

Steve Price

The Hospital Episode Statistics (HES) system provides extensive information about the inpatient treatment delivered by NHS hospitals in England. This is stored in a central database which contains annual record sets from 1989 to the present. There are similar, although separately administered, systems for Northern Ireland, Scotland and Wales. Output from HES, either in the form of summary tabulations or copies of the individual records themselves – subject to strict controls – is made available for a wide variety of uses. This is discussed further in the section on HES output (p. 61).

A unique resource

A wide variety of data conforming to national standards is collected from NHS hospitals for the purpose of central analysis and perform-ance monitoring. However, most of this is obtained as aggregate counts of patients and resources falling into predefined categories. Statistical returns covering aggregate data are discussed in Chapter 12. HES is different in that for each inpatient an individual record of care is submitted which contains wide-ranging details of the treatment delivered. Box 4.1 gives an overview of the data items which form the base HES record. These items are generated from a subset of the Admitted Patient Care (APC) dataset, which is the record of care that must be forwarded by all hospital providers (typically NHS trusts) to the relevant health authority, general practitioner and primary care group (PCG) to which the patient belongs. Locally, APC records provide information for detailed monitoring of hospital care by those organisations that are respons-ible for commissioning treatment. Prior to April 1999 the APC was used to support the operation of the NHS internal market, each record providing notification to the patient's health authority that a 'chargeable' service had been provided by the NHS trust originating the record.

The record-based nature of HES provides a very high degree of flexibility. An almost infinite variety of tabulations can be generated directly from the central database. Where it is necessary to examine individual records in detail, it is even possible to extract record sets from the database which may then be loaded on to secondary systems for further analysis and manipulation. However, because of the sensitive nature of such low level data, strict controls are in place to ensure that confidentiality is respected.

Consultant episodes

An HES record is generated for each episode of inpatient care under a particular consultant within a single hospital provider. Inpatient care includes day surgery. If responsibility for an admitted patient is passed from one consultant to another, a separate HES record must be constructed for each *consultant episode*. An example of treatment involving more than one consultant episode is where a patient is first admitted to an emergency ward for initial assessment and stabilisation under one consultant, and then transferred to a general ward for continued care under a second consultant. If a patient is transferred from one hospital provider to another – perhaps because the first hospital is not equipped to provide the highly specialised care which the patient's condition demands – at least one HES record is required from each hospital. Technically, the patient is discharged from the first hospital in order to be admitted to the second, even though their period of inpatient care is effectively continuous.

Because a given patient may be treated by a number of consultants or be transferred between hospital providers or perhaps have a number of entirely separate periods of inpatient care during a particular datayear, there could be more than one record deposited in the HES database for that patient. As the records within the HES database are not currently linked together, a degree of care must therefore be exercised in interpreting aggregate counts derived from the data. Fortunately, admission details (date of admission to hospital, method of admission and, where applicable, waiting time) are copied on to all records pertaining to a particular spell (i.e. continuous period of treatment within a single hospital provider). This makes the analysis of spells, as opposed to individual consultant episodes, entirely possible, although there are some limitations as to what can be achieved. It is even possible, using algorithms which associate and

Box 4.1 The main HES record

Admission
Date
Date decided (*elective admissions*)
Method (*elective, emergency, other*)
Source (e.g. *residential accommodation*)
Status (*psychiatric patient*)
Waiting time

Carer support indicator★

Category (*amenity, NHS, private*)

Classification (*day case, ordinary*)

Intended management★

Consultant
GMC code★
Main specialty (*provider contract*)
Treatment specialty

Diagnosis
Primary
Subsidiary
Secondary (*first 5*)

Discharge
Date
Destination (e.g. *residential accommodation*)
Method

Episode (*of care under a consultant*)
Start and end dates
Status (*finished, unfinished*)
Type (*birth, delivery, ordinary*)

General practitioner★

Neonatal level of care

Operation
First four surgical procedure codes
Date(s) of procedure(s)

Patient
Date of birth
Ethnic group
NHS number★
Postcode
Sex

Provider (e.g. *NHS trust*)
Organisation identifier
Site code★
Local Patient Identifier★
Spell number★

Purchaser or PCG code

Referrer (*consultant, GMP or GDP*)★

★Items included from the 1997/98 datayear.
Note: These items are centrally collected from all episodes of NHS inpatient care.

then sort individual records into chronological order, to analyse all details of a person's inpatient care during a particular year (*see* section on future developments, p. 62).

The HES database consists of separate annual recordsets, each covering the period from 1 April to 31 March in the following year. These periods are known as HES datayears. The recordset for a particular datayear will contain all those records relating to consultant episodes which finished within the datayear – because the patient was either discharged from hospital or transferred to another consultant or hospital provider. This gives rise to the term *finished consultant episode* (FCE). There are around 10 million separate records for each datayear, and 98% of these are FCEs. The remaining 2% of records relate to unfinished episodes, i.e. records for patients who were occupying a hospital bed at midnight on 31 March. For each unfinished episode, a partial record is constructed which facilitates limited analysis (but *see* section on supplementary data, p. 58). When the patient's treatment is completed – almost certainly during the following datayear – a record of the now *finished* consultant episode will be generated. This means that in any analysis covering a number of consecutive datayears it is important to exclude records relating to unfinished episodes, otherwise certain periods of care will be counted twice. These concepts are illustrated in Figure 4.1.

Analysis of HES data has shown that approximately 94% of all hospital spells consist of just one consultant episode.

Types of analysis

The wide-ranging nature of the data contained in each HES record (*see* Box 4.1) facilitates many different kinds of analysis. Although not comprehensive, the following points give an idea as to what may be achieved.

- The primary diagnosis, any subsidiary diagnosis and up to five secondary diagnoses are recorded. For the datayears up to, and including, 1994/95 these are coded according to the International Classification of Diseases (ICD), ninth revision. From the 1995/96 datayear, the tenth revision of ICD has been used. Counts of any one diagnosis code, or counts of cases having diagnoses falling within a specified range, or ranges, may easily be obtained. It is also possible to isolate cases where a specified combination of

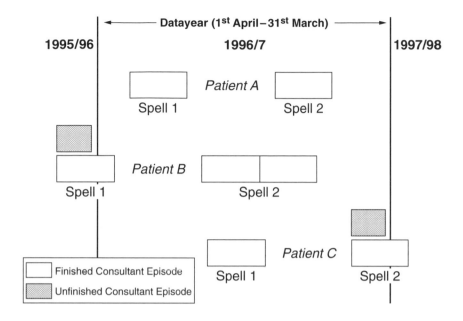

Figure 4.1 The relationship between spells and consultant episodes. Represented here are three patients who each have two spells of inpatient treatment during the period shown. Patient A is treated by one consultant during both his first and second stays in hospital, and so there are just two HES records – one for each spell. Patient B was first admitted shortly before the end of the 1995/96 datayear, but discharged during the early part of the 1996/97 datayear. Full details of Patient B's first spell of treatment are therefore recorded in the 1996/97 datayear, because that is when the episode of care finished. However, an unfinished record (shown by the shaded rectangle) is deposited in the 1995/96 datayear, and gives partial details of the episode. Patient B was readmitted to hospital later in the 1996/97 datayear and during this second spell of treatment, responsibility for care was transferred to a second consultant. Hence there are two HES records detailing Patient B's second spell. Patient C has three HES records. One for the first spell, which began and ended during the 1996/97 datayear, and two for the second spell, which also began during 1996/97, but ended when Patient C was discharged during 1997/98. Full details of spell 2 are therefore recorded in the 1997/98 datayear, but there is also an unfinished record deposited in 1996/97.

diagnoses codes exists; for example where it is necessary to ascertain the cause of a particular condition by associating a primary diagnosis with a separate code in the range V01 to Y98 under ICD10 or perhaps where there is a dagger and asterisk relationship between codes. In this latter case the 'dagger' code – a reference to the typographical symbol used in the printed classification to identify a code which may be used in this way – relates to the underlying disease, whereas the 'asterisk' code indicates a manifestation of the disease in a particular organ or site which is a clinical problem in its own right. The dagger code must always immediately precede the asterisk code and will therefore normally be the primary diagnosis.

- Up to the first four surgical procedures are recorded using the OPCS4 classification adopted for use within the UK. Summary counts of operations can therefore be provided, and it is also possible to carry out more complex analyses involving specified diagnoses (*see* above). For example, an aggregate could be produced showing the numbers of leg amputations performed where the patient was suffering from diabetes.

- The dates of admission, discharge and waiting times are recorded. This makes it possible, for example, to analyse the length of stay in hospital for patients with particular primary diagnoses. Alternatively, the waiting times for specified surgical procedures can be obtained. Use may also be made of the 'provider code' which reveals the hospital provider (in recent years an NHS trust) where the patient was treated.

- The patient's date of birth and home address postcode provide the basis for age-related and demographic analysis. In order to assist in this, and also to ensure confidentiality, a number of data items are prederived from these base items (e.g. the patient's age in a whole number of years and the health authority area where they resided).

- The broad specialty (e.g. urology) under which the patient was treated, the method of admission (emergency or from a waiting list, etc.), the method of discharge (including death of patient) and a number of more specialised factors may also be taken into account.

Although some of the more obvious associations have been alluded to above, there are actually very few restrictions on the type of analysis that may be undertaken. Table 4.1 shows an example of a tabulation produced from the HES database.

Because HES data is available for 1989/90 and all subsequent years, it is common for analyses to be requested covering a considerable time span. Although this is possible, great care must often be exercised in the interpretation of the results. For example, there have been many changes in the organisation of the NHS during the past decade. Health authority boundaries have altered considerably, and there are now far fewer health authorities covering

Table 4.1 A tabulation of HES data

1995/96 Datayear	Episodes count	Length of stay Mean	Median	Occupied bed days Sum	Waiting time Mean	Median	Patient age Mean
Operations on lung (E53–E59)	7 565	10.1	8	66 973	18.7	11	60
Operations on liver (J01–J16)	15 334	7.9	2	98 871	28.0	13	51
Replacement of coronary artery (K40–K4)	15 848	11.9	9	148 858	152.1	130	62
Abdominal branches of aorta (L41–L47)	3 552	5.5	2	16 230	29.1	17	57
Hip replacement (W37–W39)	45 954	14.2	12	628 133	192.0	161	69

Notes: These figures relate to a small selection of surgical procedures performed during the 1995/96 datayear. The relevant OPCS4 codes appear in brackets. The figures cover all hospital providers in England, but it would also have been possible to provide data separately for each NHS trust or to present the figures for a number of patient age groups, for example.

England than there were 10 years ago. Also, in the early years of HES, hospitals were managed by district health authorities and did not exist as separately identifiable entities within HES. They were later granted a degree of autonomy as directly managed units (DMUs), before finally acquiring the status of NHS trusts.

Supplementary data

A proportion of HES records have sets of additional data items appended to them which provide information about specific aspects of the episode of care, as follows.

- **Maternity**. Where the record relates to a delivery (the mother's record) or birth (the record for a baby), 19 items are appended which summarise the birth event. Note that for every birth, including those which take place outside NHS hospitals, separate HES records are compiled for both the mother and the baby. Each record carries the same set of additional items. In the case of multiple births, each baby's record has one set of additional items, whereas the mother's record will have a separate set for each baby, up to a maximum of six.

- **Psychiatric census**. Sixteen additional items are appended to the unfinished records of psychiatric patients either formally detained under specific sections of the Mental Health Act 1983 or who had remained in hospital for a year or more, and were occupying NHS hospital beds at midnight on 31 March.

- **Augmented care**. Since 1 October 1997 (i.e. from the middle of the 1997/98 datayear), 13 items have been appended to records for patients where the episode included either high dependency or intensive care.

A listing of these supplementary items is given in Box 4.2. Please note that because hospitals are often required to make special arrangements in order to collect these, the quality and completeness of the data are subject to variation.

Collection and processing

Prior to the 1996/97 datayear, the HES records generated by individual hospital providers were forwarded via the appropriate regional health authority (RHA) where they were assembled into a regional submission on either a quarterly or annual basis. The

Box 4.2 Supplementary data collected for certain groups of patients

Augmented Care (*from October 1997*)
Start date; where patient came from; location of care (unit); whether planned; specialty of management; duration of high dependency care; duration of intensive care; number of augmented care periods within episode; number of organs supported; care period number; outcome; disposal; end date.

Maternity
Length of gestation; method of inducement; method of delivery; anaesthetic during delivery; post delivery anaesthetic; method of resuscitation; birth state; birth order; sex; birth weight; date of birth (baby); date of birth (mother); status of person conducting delivery; intended delivery place; delivery place; reason for any change of delivery place; number of babies; number of previous pregnancies; first antenatal assessment date.

Psychiatric Census
Census date; diagnosis (× 7); duration of stay; age; status (whether detained); legal status; category (Mental Health Act 1983); detention date; duration of detention; ward type.

national dataset would then become available for general analysis approximately one year after the datayear had ended.

The RHAs were abolished on 1 April 1996 and from that date the responsibility for transmitting APC data and therefore, indirectly, HES records began to be transferred to the NHS wide clearing service (NWCS). The NWCS (also referred to as ClearNet) provides an electronic messaging service for the NHS, and is structured around a central hub, through which all data must pass. HES records are now obtained by quarterly extraction from a temporary store which forms part of this hub. Improvements in the speed of transmission and processing now facilitate provisional analysis of HES data shortly after the end of each quarter. However, the finalised annual datasets which provide the most accurate information do not become available until some time after the datayear has ended.

Before records are entered into the HES database they are analysed in order to check for any shortcomings in their coding. Data quality reports are fed back to hospital providers and, in extreme cases, retransmission of the data via the NWCS may be requested. Because of the numbers of records involved, much of this analysis is automated, and extends to the use of algorithms which are capable of actually correcting obvious errors. In other cases, although the algorithm may be capable of identifying an error (for example the use of a diagnosis code which does not form part of the ICD classification), corrective action must be restricted to overwriting the offending item with a value recognised as signifying that the data is not available (in the case of the primary diagnosis, the IDC10 code R69 is used). More details are given in the Department of Health publication entitled *How HES Data is Processed.*[1]

Additional data items are also added to each record in order to simplify the scripting of queries and reduce the time taken to process enquiries. These items include:

- the duration of the episode in days calculated by subtracting the start date from the end date. A similar calculation is also performed for the duration of the complete hospital stay (spell) in the case of records carrying a discharge date
- the patient's age in years at the beginning and also the end of the episode is calculated from their date of birth
- the patient's postcode is used to generate items indicating in which electoral ward, local authority district, health authority and region they lived
- healthcare resource group (HRG) codes.

Grossing

When all records for a datayear have been collected, and any possible corrections to the data have been made, an assessment is carried out in order to ascertain the completeness of the data. This partly involves comparison of the number of HES records held with an aggregate count of FCEs, known as the KP70 return, completed by every hospital provider. Also, the proportion of HES records which lack a specific primary diagnosis is ascertained.

This analysis is used to calculate specific grossing factors applicable to predefined groups of HES records (for example, all records originating from hospital providers located within the same regional office area that carry a particular set of specialty codes and have the same patient classification, i.e. either day case or ordinary admission). These factors are then written on to individual HES records so that subsequent aggregates generated from the database may be automatically weighted to account for any deficiencies in coverage and clinical data. However, where it is deemed that an unadjusted count is more appropriate for a given analysis, the grossing function may be disabled.

On-line enquiry service

Direct access to the HES database is provided for appropriate sections within the NHS Executive, including the regional offices, and the wider Department of Health. Dial-up access to HES is also being trialled in a number of other locations, including an Institute of Public Health, a university department working closely with the NHS and certain health authorities. Further details on this trial can be obtained from the Department of Health's HES Section.[1]

On-line access is restricted to the running of queries against the database for the purposes of producing aggregate counts and other summary statistics (e.g. mean length of stay for specified groups). For reasons of security and confidentiality, users are never allowed sight of individual records.

HES output

Tabulations of HES data are provided routinely for officials within the Department of Health. This information is invaluable as an aid to performance management, forward planning and the monitoring of clinical effectiveness. HES is also used to answer questions tabled by Members of Parliament.

Under the provisions of Open Government, and in line with an ongoing commitment to disseminate information about healthcare generally, health authorities, NHS trusts, public bodies, private companies and, last but not least, interested members of the public are free to make enquiries about any aspect of inpatient treatment.

In nearly all cases, tabulations providing aggregate counts are sufficient to answer the questions posed. However, in areas such as medical research it is occasionally necessary for the individual records to be examined. Needless to say, very strict controls must be exercised in these cases, and only those portions of the particular records relevant to the research will be released. In order to ensure that the necessary conditions are met, most applications for data extracts must first be scrutinised by the NWCS Security and Confidentiality Group, currently chaired by Professor Alistair Bellingham.[2]

If the requested output is a simple tabulation this may be provided free of charge, but where greater complexity is involved a charge reflecting the cost of producing the output is normally levied.

Future developments

It has long been recognised that the lack of any permanent linkage between HES records pertaining to the same patient is a drawback of the present system. It is not routinely possible, for example, to ascertain how regularly certain patients undergo hospital treatment within the span of a year, even though the database actually contains a separate and comprehensive record of each treatment.

However, it has been possible to establish temporary associations between records relating to the same patient by a process of sorting the database according to data items which help identify individuals – primarily date of birth, sex and postcode. This has, for example, allowed the analysis of emergency readmissions to hospital.

From the 1997/98 datayear, the new NHS number was added to HES records. This greatly assists in the matching of records relating to the same patient, and has provided the impetus to exploit further the possibilities of record linkage. It has, therefore, been decided that in future, HES records will be enhanced by the addition of items which reveal something about any other periods of inpatient treatment during the same year. These additions, known collectively as the In Year Patient Record (IYPR), will go some way towards making HES a patient-based system.

Looking further ahead there is the possibility that HES data may be made more widely available using technologies such as the Internet. The broadening of the user base in such ways will further help to justify the not inconsiderable cost of collecting the data.

References

1   Department of Health Hospital Episode Statistics Section (published annually) *How HES Data is Processed*. Hospital Episodes Statistics Section, Statistics Division, Department of Health, London. (Available free on request from: Department of Health, HES Section, Room 430B, Skipton House, 80 London Road, London SE1 6LH. Tel: 020–7972–5683, Fax: 020–7972–5662, E-mail: sd2hes@doh.gov.uk)

2   Department of Health Hospital Episode Statistics Section (revised periodically) *Specifying Extracts and Tabulations from the Hospital Episode Statistics Database*. Hospital Episodes Statistics Section, Statistics Division, Department of Health, London. (Available free on request.)

5 Primary care

Deana Leadbeter

Introduction

This chapter considers official statistics in the context of primary care, and discusses data sources and a variety of possible uses. The chapter considers what the data collected at primary care level have to offer the NHS as a whole. The needs of primary care groups (PCGs), and the information available to them, are discussed but, since PCGs were only introduced on 1 April 1999 there is, at the time of writing, still much work to do to understand the information available, and needed, at primary care level.

Information available at primary care level

There is a range of information currently available regarding healthcare at the primary care level and the main data sources are discussed below. Information from these primary care sources is of use at all levels of the healthcare system, not just within primary care.

Information from general practice

At the time of writing full access to information derived from data on GP systems is not possible. However, some information is available, and the rapid increase in computerisation within GP practices provides opportunities for accessing and exchanging information electronically. A conference organised by the Health Statistics Users Group (HSUG) in 1995 considered the issue of what information general practice could deliver for measuring morbidity and health,[1] and pilot projects on accessing morbidity data from GP systems for health needs assessment and monitoring were discussed, as well as national databases.

National general practice databases
National databases include the National Morbidity Studies in General Practice, undertaken by the ONS in conjunction with the

Royal College of General Practitioners at 10-year intervals,[2,3] which are discussed in more detail in the section on general practice records in Chapter 3.

The largest national database of GP records is the General Practice Research Database (GPRD),[4-10] which has passed from its creator, VAMP Ltd, to Reuters. Reuters donated the GPRD to the Department of Health in 1994. The Office for National Statistics (formerly OPCS) operated the database from 1994 to 1999, and the Medicines Control Agency has been responsible for its overall management and financial control since April 1999. The GPRD has collected data from 1989 to date, via several versions of software supplied by InPS (formerly VAMP), from 400 to 500 practices, involving more than 6 million patients.

This large and versatile dataset has been used extensively in drug safety and efficacy studies, in disease epidemiology using case control and cohort designs and is increasingly used for health economics and outcomes work. It has also been used as a survey sampling frame.

The GPRD requires its contributors (who are paid for their data) to record their clinical data to a specified research standard. This includes ensuring complete data on registration, pregnancy, births and deaths, as well as specifying standards for the recording of diagnostic, preventive and therapeutic activity. It also specifies the handling of information between the GP, hospitals and other healthcare agencies. Feedback on data quality is given after every 6-weekly collection from the practices and includes individual vital events records for correction.

Access to the GPRD requires funds to meet the data access and extraction charges. The approval of the GPRD's Scientific and Ethical Advisory Group is also required. It should be noted that data from this large and complex dataset requires a range of skills in its use and interpretation.[11] The relevant clinical, computing and statistical skills for each research question must be employed along with an understanding of the healthcare delivery changes in which GPs have practised over the past 10 years.

Enquiries about the GPRD should be made to the Medicines Control Agency on 020–7373–0206. Enquiries for data access from academic and government bodies may also be made to the General Practice Research Team at the ONS on 020-7533-5118.

Collection of Health Data from General Practice

The Collection of Health Data from General Practice (CHDGP) project was set up in 1996 as one of the facilitating projects within the NHS Executive Information Management and Technology (IM&T) Strategy.[12] The aim was to facilitate setting up local data collection schemes, to avoid unnecessary duplication, and to ensure that data collected are comparable between practices. This last issue of ensuring comparability was highlighted in the 1995 HSUG conference[1] as one of the main difficulties in bringing data together across practices. The CHDGP project also aimed to encourage the development of standard software called MIQUEST to provide a standard method for expressing queries and extracting data with proper safeguards and controls. The MIQUEST approach allows for the collection of aggregated or anonymised data from general practice computer systems. It is a non-proprietary specification of: a structured health query language (HQL) which is a health-specific variant of SQL; query and response file formats; and EDIFACT messages. It incorporates safeguards against unauthorised and inappropriate access to patient data, which have been checked with the Royal Colleges and the BMA.

A two-year pilot project period ended in March 1999. During this period the CHDGP project continued to:

- support and encourage the use of patient health data held in GP systems
- provide practical help to improve data quality
- develop guidelines and training programmes
- support and develop MIQUEST data extraction software and methods
- test the value of comparative analysis across GP practices
- work with volunteers in more than 20 pilot schemes covering around 200 practices
- provide a comparative analysis service.

Sets of MIQUEST queries have been tested for: heart disease; hypertension; diabetes; cerebrovascular disease; severe mental illness; asthma; and risk factors; as well as for basic data. The pilot phase initially concentrated on obtaining data from EMIS and Meditel GP systems but developments are under way, or completed, to allow the use of MIQUEST on a further seven commonly used GP computer systems.

Examples of the queries run by the Comparative Analysis Service (CAS) during the pilot period are given in Table 5.1. These data have been useful in helping to formulate early thoughts on the usage of data in PCGs.

Table 5.1 Examples of queries run by the CHDGP Comparative Analysis Service

Adult patients with asthma who have a peak flow reading <150 in the last year

Patients with asthma who have been seen for asthma in the last year

Patients with diabetes with co-morbidities: hypertensive disease or ischaemic heart disease

Patients with diabetes who have a record of HbA1c within the last year, analysed by good, moderate and poor control values

Patients with hypertension who have a record of blood pressure taken within the last year, and mean of the last three readings (whenever taken) analysed by above or below 160/90

Patients with hypertension who smoke and with a record of smoking advice

Patients with hypertension with a record of alcohol consumption

Patients with CVA who have a record of serum cholesterol ever

Patients with CVA who have a record of aspirin prescription or aspirin advice; have a record of aspirin allergy

Patients with IHD with a record of diet advice; exercise advice

Patients with hypertension with a record of medication, analysed by drug group

Patients with TIA *without* CVA (these patients can then be reviewed and possibly offered more aggressive treatment)

Patients for whom diagnostic codes are not being used but have mental illness-associated codes in their record (e.g. referral to psychiatry, use of specific drugs)

Patients who are taking statins who have a record of diabetes, IHD, CVA, hypertension.

All patients who have a record of alcohol consumption; consume more than recommended levels

Although the pilot period has ended it is planned that training and support will continue. It is also planned that a flexible comparative analysis service will continue to be offered, with PCGs being able to select from query sets and report formats on a variety of topics.

All the reference documentation for the CHDGP project, latest news on the availability of services, and details of contacts in participating local schemes (many of whom have produced their own guidelines and reports) are available from the project website at http://www.nottingham.ac.uk/chdgp/ or from the project support team in the NHS Executive on 0113-254-6024, who also hold supplies of publications on the project. For more detailed advice, the CHDGP training and support team (based at Nottingham University) can be contacted on 0115-919-4495.

Other primary care systems

In addition to the general practice systems there are a range of other national computer systems relating to the primary care sector which can potentially produce national statistics. The British Computer Society handbook on primary care systems,[13] in the *Information Management in Health Care* series of handbooks, provides an overview of these systems. This includes the Exeter core systems covering screening (discussed further below), patient registration and the NHS Central Register. A more up to date picture of the current Exeter systems can be obtained from the NHS Information Authority's website at http://www.exeter.nhsia.nhs.uk/. The website describes each system and the statistics that can be produced from it. The statistics listed include the statutory returns that are provided from the system to the Department of Health, and which are then available from the Department of Health (*see* Chapter 12 for a more detailed discussion of statutory returns in general).

Cervical and breast screening programmes

The Department of Health series of Statistical Bulletins includes bulletins on the cervical screening programme[14] and on the breast screening programme.[15] The bulletin on the cervical screening programme summarises information for England from the computerised call and recall system for cervical screening (collected on return KC53) and information about cervical smears examined at pathology laboratories (collected on return KC61, which includes some information about symptomatic as well as screening programme smears). The bulletin provides information about the coverage of the screening programme and about the test results. The information given is analysed by age, by region and by health authority. The bulletin on the breast screening programme summarises information for England from the breast screening units about the operation and the outcomes of the call and recall system for breast cancer screening (collected on return KC62). It also includes information from health authorities about the population coverage of the programme (collected on return KC63). The information given is analysed by age, by region and by health authority. These bulletins are updated annually and a listing of the bulletins and statistics currently available is given on the Department of Health's website (http://www.doh.gov.uk/).

Information about GPs

The Department of Health series of Statistical Bulletins includes a bulletin summarising the statistics on general medical practitioners in England from 1988 to 1998.[16] This looks at the changes during this period in GPs and in GP practices. The changes reviewed include:

- number, type and sex of GP
- distribution of doctors by age, and by partnership size
- average list sizes
- contractual commitments of GPs (full time, part time, job share)
- practice staff employed
- services provided to patients.

In addition to the information routinely available on GPs, the Department of Health carried out two surveys in April and May 1999 in England on access to GPs and GP clinics, and access to community-based clinics out of office hours.[17]

Another useful source of information about GPs and GP practices is the Medical Practices Committee (MPC). The MPC aims to ensure that GPs are equitably distributed throughout England and Wales in accordance with the healthcare needs of the population. Their annual report for 1997/98 reviews the current situation and is based not only on routine data on GPs but also on a survey of GP recruitment and retirement, which they carry out each year.[18,19] Further information on the work of the MPC can be obtained via their website (http://www.open.gov.uk/doh/mpc/mpch.htm).

Pharmaceutical data

Information on pharmacies, and on prescribing and dispensing, can be used for several purposes. Community pharmacists provide an important service within the NHS, not only dispensing prescriptions, but also providing an easily accessible service of advice and over-the-counter treatment, which complements the work of GPs. Information on the availability of community pharmacy services is therefore important for planning healthcare service delivery at the primary care level. Information on the actual drugs prescribed and dispensed is also of use. Monitoring prescribing patterns provides information to assist in improving the appropriateness and cost effectiveness of prescribing. In addition, where information on the incidence of particular diseases or conditions is not easily available from other sources, prescription information can be used as a proxy measure for disease or condition incidence.

Prescribing information

Information on prescribing can be obtained from the Prescription Pricing Authority (PPA), although the information they hold is not in the public domain and is, in general, only made available within the NHS. The PPA is a special health authority within the National Health Service Executive (NHSE) and one of its functions is the provision of prescribing and dispensing information to the NHS (excluding hospital dispensing). Information is provided in a variety of formats to the Department of Health (DoH), NHSE, regional offices of the NHSE (ROs), health authorities (HAs), hospitals, medical and pharmaceutical advisers, NHS trusts, dispensers, police, auditors, Home Office and research groups.

There are four major information systems that provide a broad spectrum of prescribing information.

- Prescribing analysis and cost (**PACT**). PACT standard reports provide GPs with reliable and regular information on their prescribing habits and costs on a quarterly basis. The reports give number of prescriptions, the 20 leading cost drugs, the top 40 British National Formulary (BNF) sections and the average cost per prescription. In addition to the standard reports a different drug-related issue is discussed each quarter.
- Indicative prescribing scheme (**IPS**). IPS provides information to GPs, health authorities, regional offices, and the Department of Health on prescribing costs against prescribing budgets.
- Prescribing cost analysis (**PCA**). The PCA system provides national drug information to the Department of Health and covers:
  - drug analysis (summary data on costs and number of items dispensed)
  - pharmacy analysis (summary data on number, size and type of pharmacies)
  - dispensing doctor analysis (summary data on number and costs of prescriptions written by dispensing doctors).
- Electronic PACT (**ePACT**). This provides standard PACT reports on a monthly basis, and also provides facilities for the

data to be compared, for example between different types of practices, and then presented in a number of different formats.

Further information can be obtained from the PPA's website at http://www.ppa.org.uk.

Another useful source for general information about prescribing is the National Prescribing Centre (NPC). The NPC is a health service organisation, formed in April 1996 by the NHS Executive, following a review of centrally funded support for prescribing and medicine use. The NPC's current aim is 'to facilitate the promotion of high quality, cost-effective prescribing through a coordinated and prioritised programme of activities aimed at supporting all relevant professionals and senior managers working in the new NHS'. The aims of the NPC's programme include helping to meet the demands of health improvement programmes (HImPs) and of PCGs. Further information on the activities of the NPC can be obtained from its website on http://www.npc.co.uk.

Community pharmacies

In addition to the information on prescriptions available from the PPA, the Department of Health produces 6-monthly bulletins which present information about community pharmacies in contract with HAs in England and Wales to dispense NHS prescriptions.[20] The Department of Health has also produced a bulletin which presents similar information over the period 1990/91 to 1998/99.[21] These bulletins also provide information about openings and closures of such contractors, decisions on applications in connection with such contracts and schemes for the disposal of unwanted medicines.

Survey of NHS patients

In the White Paper *The New NHS: modern, dependable*,[22] the Department of Health is committed to improving quality of care and to reducing inequalities in performance practice. One element of these reforms is to carry out a programme of national surveys looking at patient experience. The 1998 General Practice Survey[23] was the first in this programme of national surveys.

A sample of people in each of the 100 health authorities in England was surveyed and covered a wide range of issues including:

- access and waiting times
- communication between patients and GPs

- patients' views of GPs' knowledge
- out-of-hours care
- competence and courtesy
- helpfulness and availability of other surgery staff and services, including practice nurses and receptionists.

Other primary care data

Lists of statistics and publications available from the Department of Health can be found on their website (http://www.doh.gov.uk/public/stats3.htm for statistics and http://www.doh.gov.uk/public/hpsspub.htm for publications). In addition to the primary care data discussed in this chapter other statistics and reports relating to primary care are available, including information on many other services such as contraceptive and immunisation services, general ophthalmic services, chiropody services and a variety of other community health services.

Recent developments in primary care

In considering both the future of information available from primary care, and the information needs at the primary care level, it is important to consider how primary care, as a whole, is developing.

In Chapter 5 of the White Paper *The New NHS: modern, dependable*, published in December 1997,[22] and in the subsequent Health Act of 1999,[24] proposals for the development of primary and community healthcare in England were put forward. It is the current government's stated intention to place primary care at the heart of its programme to modernise the health service and a key feature of these proposals is the establishment of primary care groups (PCGs).[25,26] The proposals were seen as building on successful, recent developments in primary care. These developments included an increased role for GPs, or groups of GPs, in commissioning and contracting for services, and also an extension of the range of services provided within individual surgeries. The developments followed on from the introduction of GP fundholding in the NHS and Community Care Act in 1990,[27] and the personal medical services pilot schemes introduced in the NHS Primary Care Act in 1997.[28]

In addition to the focus on a primary care-led NHS there has been an increased emphasis in the NHS on looking at the health of the population, instead of just at the health services delivered. A White Paper *Health of the Nation*, published in July 1992,[29,30] was followed in February 1998 with the consultative document *Our Healthier Nation*,[31] and in July 1999 with the White Paper *Saving Lives: our healthier nation*.[32] This emphasis on health, rather than health services, has led to a greater understanding that many of the activities and interventions that affect the population's health occur at a primary care level, and that information about some of these activities is only available through primary care level information systems

Information needs at primary care level

The focus on a primary care-led NHS, with the development of PCGs and an increasing role of GPs in commissioning and contracting, has meant changes to the information needs at primary care level. The official statistics available on health and health services need to be reviewed to see how well they meet these new needs, and much work is being carried out on this at the time of writing. This chapter can only give an indication of the direction in which this work is going. It is expected that, over the next year or so, this work will develop further.

In developing information strategies for primary care, and for PCGs in particular, an understanding is required, at both local and national level, of what kind of information and infrastructure is needed so that PCGs can impact on the health of local people. This involves considering the roles of PCGs, the information needs arising from these roles, and the issues involved in meeting these needs. In terms of the focus of this book this needs to include consideration of what official statistics are available that can help to meet these information needs. The discussion that follows on the information needs of PCGs draws on the output from a day conference on *Information for PCGs* on 12 March 1999, which was arranged by the national HSUG.[33]

Why do PCGs need information?

PCGs began operating from April 1999 and their key functions are:

- to improve the health of, and address health inequality in, the local community
- to develop primary and community health services by improving

the quality of those services, and dealing with poor performance in primary care providers

- to commission services for their patients from NHS hospital trusts.

Some of the tasks that need to be carried out in order to fulfil these roles include:

- assessing population needs
- monitoring health status
- planning health services
- contract monitoring
- budget management
- feedback of information to practices
- public accountability and clinical governance.

All of these tasks depend on relevant, up to date and accurate information being available to PCGs and primary care practitioners. They require a range of information to carry out these tasks – both 'hard' and 'soft' data – and they need to use official/national statistics, as well as statistics from many other sources. Information that is currently available from official sources to assist in these tasks includes:

- population estimates
- vital statistics – births, deaths, cancer
- socio-economic information
- health services data – referrals, admissions, prescribing, community health services.

General issues with regard to the availability and use of much of this information have been discussed elsewhere in this book: socio-economic information is discussed in Chapter 1, mortality data in Chapter 2, population data in Chapter 3, hospital activity data in Chapter 4, births data in Chapter 9 and cancer data in Chapter 10. There are, however, some specific issues in relation to using these general data sources to support the work of PCGs, and these are considered below.

PCG populations

Census data and population estimates are available from the Office for National Statistics (ONS). An issue that arises when using these data to support the work of PCGs is that, traditionally, ONS and NHS information systems, and also other relevant agencies such as Social Services, have generated mainly area-based data. However, PCGs will be practice based, although with an 'area' commitment. GP practices do not follow defined boundaries and, since PCGs are defined in terms of practices, they also do not follow defined boundaries. It is, therefore, currently difficult to obtain population information for PCGs and hence to calculate rates for PCG activity.

PCGs have a dual responsibility – to the population in a geographical area, as well as to their practice lists. This leads to different possible definitions of PCG populations, resulting in the possibility that population bases may vary according to which PCG activity is being examined. Possible ways of defining the population for a particular PCG are, for example:

- patients on the lists of the GPs within the PCG wherever the patients live
- patients on the lists of the GPs within the PCG where the patients live in a defined area
- population estimates for a defined area.

Another problem to be addressed is reconciling population estimates based on GP lists with those from the ONS. In 1999 it was reported that, nationally, there was a 3% difference between the ONS and GP-list estimates of resident population. However, the difference varies considerably between regions, from 1% to 10%, and also varies between health authorities within regions.

Initially, resource allocation for PCGs will be based on historic spend, although it will eventually be based on a formula which will take into account the age structure of the population, deprivation and mortality variables. The issue of determining the population of a PCG is therefore crucial for budget allocation.

Vital statistics and socio-economic data

These data are discussed in Chapters 2 and 3, and cancer statistics are discussed in Chapter 10. The same problem arises as with population estimates when using these data for PCGs, since vital statistics and socio-economic data are traditionally area based. It is understood that the ONS is considering adding PCG codes to the central postcode directory, which will allow for the production of rates for specific events by PCG areas. However, the production of event rates for PCG populations is more difficult, as has already been mentioned. For socio-economic data the NHSE has produced the Attribution Data Set. This links patients on GP lists to enumeration districts, and can be used to generate proxy census variables for PCGs.

NHS hospital activity data

Hospital Episode Statistics (HES) in general are covered in Chapter 4. HES, however, only covers admitted patient care. Data on outpatient referrals and Accident & Emergency Department attendances, although likely to be available to PCGs from local NHS trusts, are currently not easily available on national databases.

In order to use the information held in NHS activity databases to support the work of PCGs, it is important that the GP practice code is available, and that it is completely and accurately recorded. Although this is currently a problem it is hoped that the development of PCGs, and hence the increased importance of this data item, will lead to improvements in future.

Also, as has already been mentioned, the PCG boundaries are related to patients on GP lists instead of being area based. Some patients on a GP's list may well reside in a different health authority than the one in which the GP's PCG is based. The current national arrangements for flow of data from NHS trust to the health authorities purchasing the care, the ClearNet service, are based on a patient's area of residence. This means that it can currently be difficult to obtain information on patients who live in other authorities. At present this means that data sharing is needed between health authorities, which can require a high level of commitment from the Chief Executive of the authorities involved. It is expected that, in the longer term, amendments will be made to the arrangements for flow of data to meet the needs of PCGs.

Conclusion

In this chapter the current situation with regard to statistics available from, and needed by, PCGs and primary care practitioners has been described. Of necessity the situation described in some areas is unclear since, at the time of writing, discussions and developments are still under way in relation to meeting the needs of the New NHS and of PCGs in particular.

The focus of the chapter has been on the official statistics potentially available at the primary care level, and also on the official statistics available to PCGs. Other information issues of importance at the primary care level, such as the area of information for patients and also the development of professional knowledge for primary care practitioners, have not been covered in this chapter. These are discussed in the NHSE's *Primary Care: the future*[34] and the White Paper *Primary Care: delivering the future.*[35] Proposals for meeting these needs are also put forward on the NHS Information Strategy *Information for Health.*[36,37]

Finally, in such a rapidly changing field, anyone wishing to make use of official statistics is advised to check the websites recommended for the current position with regard to the availability of data, and also with regard to the current situation on the completeness, accuracy and definitional issues that have been discussed in this chapter.

Acknowledgements

Thanks are due to the speakers at the HSUG conference held in March 1999 on *Information for PCGs*, in particular Azeem Majeed and David Gearing whose presentations have provided some of the background information for this chapter.

References

1   Health Statistics User Group (1996) *Measuring Morbidity and Health – What Information can General Practice Deliver?* Health Statistics User Group (available from dml@ftech.co.uk).

2   Hollowell J (1997) The General Practice Research Database: quality of morbidity data. *Population Trends.* 87: 36–40.

3   ONS (1998) *Key Health Statistics from General Practice.* Office for National Statistics, London.

4   General Register Office (1958) *Morbidity Statistics from General Practice, 1955–6 (Vols I–III).* Studies on Medical and Population Subjects No. 14. HMSO, London.

5   RCGP, OPCS and DoH (1974) *Morbidity Statistics from General Practice: second national study, 1970–71.* Studies on Medical and Population Subjects No. 26. HMSO, London.

6   RCGP, OPCS and DoH (1979) *Morbidity Statistics from General Practice, 1971–72: second national study.* Studies on Medical and Population Subjects No. 36. HMSO, London.

7   RCGP, OPCS and DoH (1982) *Morbidity Statistics from General Practice, 1970–71: socio-economic analysis.* Studies on Medical and Population Subjects No. 46. HMSO, London.

8   RCGP, OPCS and DoH (1986*) Morbidity Statistics from General Practice: third national study, 1981–82.* Series MB5 No. 1. HMSO, London.

9   RCGP, OPCS and DoH (1990) *Morbidity Statistics from General Practice. Third morbidity study: socioeconomic analysis 1981–82.* Series MB5 No. 2. HMSO, London.

10 McCormick A, Fleming D and Charlton J (1995) *Morbidity Statistics from General Practice: fourth national study, 1991–92.* Series MB5 No. 3. HMSO, London.

11 Lawrenson R, Williams T and Farmer R (1999) Clinical information for research; the use of general practice databases. *Journal of Public Health Medicine.* **21**(3): 299–304.

12 NHS Executive (1996) *Collection of Health Data from General Practice.* Information Management Group of the NHS Executive, Leeds.

13 Abbott W, Bryant J and Bainbridge M (eds) (1996) *Information Management in Healthcare: Handbook C Primary Care.* Health Informatics Specialist Groups (HISG) of the British Computer Society, Eastbourne.

14 Department of Health (1999) *Cervical Screening Programme, England: 1998–99.* Statistical Bulletin 1999/32 (obtainable on www.doh.gov.uk/public/sb9932.htm).

15 Department of Health (1999) *Breast Screening Programme, England: 1997–98.* Statistical Bulletin 1999/9 (obtainable on www.doh.gov.uk/public/bcscreen.htm).

16 Department of Health (1999) *Statistics for General Medical Practitioners in England: 1988–1998.* Statistical Bulletin 1999/13 (obtainable on www.doh.gov.uk/public/medprac88–98.htm).

17 Department of Health (1999*) Access to GPs and Clinics Services Out-of-Office Hours: England 1999.* Department of Health, London.

18 Medical Practices Committee (1998) *Annual Report for 1997/98.* Medical Practices Committee, London (obtainable on www.open.gov.uk/doh/mpc/mpch.htm).

19 Medical Practices Committee (1998) *Survey of GP Recruitment in England and Wales: 1998.* Medical Practices Committee, London (obtainable on www.open.gov.uk/doh/mpc/mpch.htm).

20 Department of Health (1999) *General Pharmaceutical Services in Community Pharmacies in England and Wales: 31 March 1999.* Statistical Bulletin 1999/20 (obtainable on www.doh.gov.uk/public/community-pharmacies99.htm).

21 Department of Health (1999) *Community Pharmacies in England and*

Wales: 31 March 1999. Statistical Bulletin 1999/20 (obtainable on www.doh.gov.uk/public/community-pharmacies99.htm).
22 Department of Health (1997) *The New NHS: modern, dependable.* Cmd 3807. The Stationery Office, London.
23 Department of Health (1999) *The National Survey of NHS Patients – General Practice: 1998.* Department of Health, London (obtainable on www.doh.gov.uk/public/gpnhsurvey.htm).
24 *Health Act 1999.* (Chapter c.8)
25 NHS Executive (1998) *Establishing Primary Care Groups.* Health Service Circular HSC 98/065. NHSE, Leeds.
26 NHS Executive (1998) *Developing Primary Care Groups.* Health Service Circular HSC 98/139. NHSE, Leeds.
27 *National Health Service and Community Care Act 1990.* (Chapter 19.)
28 *National Health Service (Primary Care) Act 1997.* (Chapter 46.)
29 Department of Health (1991) *Health of the Nation: a consultative document for health in England.* Cmd 1523. HMSO, London.
30 Department of Health (1992) *Health of the Nation: a strategy for health in England.* Cmd 1986. HMSO, London.
31 Department of Health (1998) *Our Healthier Nation: a contract for health.* Cmd 3852. The Stationery Office, London.
32 Department of Health (1999) *Saving Lives: our healthier nation.* Cmd 4386. The Stationery Office, London.
33 Health Statistics User Group (1999) *PCGs and their Populations: what health information is needed?* Health Statistics User Group (available from dml@ftech.co.uk).
34 NHS Executive (1996) *Primary Care: the future.* NHSE, Leeds.
35 Department of Health (1996) *Primary Care: delivering the future.* Cmd 3512. The Stationery Office, London.
36 NHS Executive (1998) *Information for Health: an information strategy for the modern NHS 1998–2005.* NHSE, Leeds.
37 NHS Executive (1998) *Information for Health: initial local implementation strategies.* NHSE, Leeds.

6 Surveying the nation's health: access to health statistics from the Data Archive

Sheila Anderson

Introduction

This chapter will describe the role and functions of the UK Data Archive. It looks at sources of data, quality control issues, and the uses to which data are put. It explains how researchers may access the Archive and gives a glimpse of rapidly developing new technology and services.

Health researchers frequently require access to official statistics, to surveys and to other sources of data and related information on health if they are to undertake meaningful research, to influence policy decisions, and to add to the body of knowledge on health issues. Important research on the relationship between diet and health and between income and health, on the effects of smoking, on the impact of sexual behaviour and on the effectiveness of advertising campaigns on the spread of AIDS, for example, could only occur because suitable data resources were available. Health researchers, then, are significant creators and users of information which, through a process of analysis, interpretation and the expertise of the researcher, is turned into knowledge. This in turn further enhances our understanding of crucial social and policy-related issues.

However, data collection is expensive and time consuming and frequently not a viable option for many researchers. Instead, many researchers turn to the existing body of survey and statistical data that has already been collected. Government departments conduct surveys and collect administrative information, and research institutions conduct surveys and collect information on a wide range of topics, much of which is of interest to health researchers. Rarely are these data resources exploited fully by the primary data collectors, leaving a rich and diverse source of information to be analysed. However, before this can occur, health researchers must first locate

information about potential resources, obtain access to those resources, and be able to use them easily and effectively. It is the role of
a data archive to facilitate this process and to provide efficient and
speedy access to data resources.

The UK Data Archive

The Data Archive (DA) at the University of Essex houses the largest
collection of accessible computer-readable social science data resources in the UK. It is a national resource centre, acquiring and
disseminating data throughout the UK and, by arrangement with
other national archives, internationally. The DA has been in existence for over 30 years and has built up an extensive collection of
social and economic statistical material, including historical material.
The collection has developed over the years to include much data of
relevance for health studies.

The functions of the DA are to:

- maintain its collection of datasets
- locate sources of data, and negotiate for their inclusion in the
  archive
- undertake quality control, validating the data, checking the
  content and provenance of data held
- disseminate data by arrangement with other national archives, and
  internationally
- help potential users to locate material of interest
- provide researchers with efficient and speedy access to data
  resources in a usable format
- regulate access to the data resources within a proper legal
  framework
- prepare data for secondary analysis.

Data collection is expensive and time consuming. By drawing on
data from an archive, researchers can concentrate more effectively on
the analysis and interpretation of relevant information.

Support for researchers

There are a number of barriers facing the potential secondary analyst
before they can successfully use data resources. They need to:

- be able to locate relevant data resources

- make sure they can obtain access to them for their intended purpose
- understand the origin and content of the source data – how and why it was collected
- be able to trust the reliability of the data, and assess any possible bias within it
- use the data in the software package of their choice on their desktop computer.

In making its data and services available the DA removes much of this burden from researchers, ensuring that they can gain access to the resources they need for their work.

Sources of health statistics

The DA holds much data of interest for health researchers, many from official sources and others from major collections created within research institutions. Data are held covering a broad range of topics in health, health services and medical care, nutrition, morbidity and mortality, accidents and injuries, fitness and exercise, drug abuse, alcohol and smoking, childbearing, family planning and abortion. Most of the data relates to the UK, but there is also international material suitable for comparative research. The major strength of the DA is that it holds social as well as direct health data, enabling social variables to be tested for their impact on health.

Leading datasets for health research available from the DA

A total of 302 datasets have health or health-related topics as the main component of their content. Below is a brief summary of some that readers of this book may find useful, including a selection of less obvious datasets. An overview of ONS surveys is given in Chapter 3.

1. Health Surveys for England and the Infant Feeding Surveys (Department of Health). Further information on the Health Survey for England is included in Chapter 7.
2. Scottish Health Surveys (Scottish Office, Department of Health).
3. General Household Survey (GHS) 1971 to present (Office of National Statistics). The General Household Survey is a multi-purpose survey, providing information on housing, employment,

education, health and social services, transport, population and social security. It is a continuous survey based on a sample of about 9000 households. Health topics fall broadly into four parts, covering activity limitation caused by sickness, consultations with the doctor, use of certain health and personal social services and visits to hospitals. Also included is use of cigarettes, use of medicines and leisure activity.

4   National Child Development Survey (NCDS), 1958 and continuing. The National Child Development Survey is a continuing longitudinal study which seeks to follow the lives of all those living in Great Britain who were born between 5 and 9 March 1958. The aim is to improve understanding of the factors affecting human development over the entire lifespan including a wide range of information on health and health-related issues. The survey is unique in following a group of people from birth, thereby offering the opportunity to track the impact of various childhood factors on adult health, tracking childhood illness and health problems, and assessing changes in health over the life course.

5   The British Household Panel Survey (BHPS), carried out by the Institute for Social and Economic Research at the University of Essex, is also a rich source of data for health research. The BHPS was designed as an annual survey of each adult (16+) member of a nationally representative sample of more than 5000 households, making a total of approximately 10 000 individual interviews. There is also a special survey of 11–15-year-old household members in the fourth cohort. Information is collected on the following topics: neighbourhood; individual demographics; residential mobility; health and caring; current employment and earnings; employment changes over the past year; lifetime childbirth, marital and relationship history; employment status history; values and opinions; household finances and organisation.

6   British Social Attitudes Surveys. These are designed to produce annual measures of attitudes which complement other large-scale government surveys. One of its main purposes is to allow the monitoring of patterns of continuity and change, and changes in attitudes in respect of a range of social issues. Questions are asked on a regular basis about welfare, health and healthcare.

7   Health Education Monitoring Survey (HEMS), 1995. The purpose of this survey was to provide a baseline measure of a set of health promotion indicators relating to health-related knowledge, attitudes and behaviour (which were developed by the Health Education Authority) of a sample of adults aged 16–74. The aim of subsequent surveys is to measure any change against this baseline.

8   Health and Lifestyle Surveys (HALS). The aim of this survey was to examine the distribution of, and the relationship between, physical and mental health, health-related behaviour (diet, exercise, smoking and alcohol consumption), social circumstances, and beliefs and attitudes, in a representative sample of the population of England, Wales and Scotland. A follow-up dataset links deaths and causes of death with the original HALS respondents.

9   Anthropometric data on children in the early twentieth century.

10 Height and weight of adults in Great Britain, 1980.

11 Height and weight data of eighteenth century army and navy recruits.

12 Youth surveys.

13 Surveys of homeless people.

14 British Crime Surveys (Home Office).

15 Eurobarometer surveys, with modules on
    – cancer and smoking
    – health and the elderly
    – immigrants and health.

Data uses

With such a large amount of data derived from different surveys the potential for research is very great. Much of the work carried out by secondary users of the data is policy driven – both informing the development of national policy and monitoring the impact of health education measures. Studies can be:

• comparative – between countries or populations
• testing associations between specific variables
• longitudinal – identifying trends
• qualitative as well as quantitative.

Examples of current research

Health Survey for England

Using the Health Survey for England, research is currently under way to:

- assess the relationship between stress and masculinity and to examine the psychosocial health of men on low income
- look at the use of health and social services and the association with measures of need and examine socio-economic differences in the use of health and social services
- compare local data with national information. For example, a project in Somerset is comparing various Somerset survey information with national figures
- understand the dynamics of age, gender and ethnicity in health and lifestyles
- assess social resources, health and disability in the population aged 55 and over
- investigate accidents in the home
- assess health expectations and access to elective care
- carry out a human health study into the health of people living in a local area
- study ill-health retirement of NHS staff
- look at the prevalence of smoking, drinking and ethnic minorities
- investigate the relationship between multiple sclerosis and general health
- investigate the relationship between ethnicity and health of older people.

General Household Survey

The General Household Survey (GHS) has been used to look at a variety of health-related research issues including:

- inequalities in health between genders, between ages and between ethnic groups
- chronic illness over the life course
- the relationship between education, economic prosperity and health

- the need for care at home
- trends in contraception
- smoking and drinking by social class
- carers and health; unemployment and health; and community care.

The Department of Health has also sponsored the ONS (the creators of the GHS) to undertake follow-up surveys of the health of people aged 65 and over, thus providing an excellent resource for examining the health and lifestyles of the elderly.

National Child Development Survey

The National Child Development Survey has been used to research:

- factors associated with changes in smoking behaviour
- modification of micturition behaviour with ageing
- *in utero* exposure to tobacco smoke and declining fertility
- childhood antecedents of psychological health differentials in a changing social context
- the history of asthma in childhood
- health and social mobility during the early years of life
- social class changes in weight for height between childhood and early adulthood
- marital selection and differences in health between married and divorced people
- childhood and early adulthood determinants of overweight status at age 33.

Scottish Health Survey

The 1995 Scottish Health Survey is the first of a series of surveys designed to make a major contribution to monitoring progress towards the health targets set out in 1991 in *Health Education in Scotland: a national policy statement* and towards the dietary targets announced in 1994. It also allows for comparative research with the Health Survey for England. For example, researchers are currently investigating:

- variations in smoking habits and smoke intake and their relation to socio-economic factors and to measures of smoke intake

- prevention of coronary heart disease in Scotland. This work replicates work already undertaken by Ramsay, using the Health Survey for England.

Combination of datasets

The data held by the archive may also be used in combination with other datasets to examine trends over time. For example, the Heights and Weights of Adults in Great Britain (1980), the Health and Lifestyle Surveys (1984/5 and 1991/2) and the Health Survey for England 1996 are being used to examine cohort trends in weight changes over a 16-year period and to offer some estimate of the future obesity status of the British population. The research group hope to identify population groups at high risk of obesity, and assess the need for obesity prevention.

British Social Attitudes Survey

Other, less obvious sources also contain data that may be of interest for health research. For example, the British Social Attitudes Surveys is being used to investigate:

- attitudes to the provision of welfare, including health services
- the demand for private healthcare services
- attitudes between private healthcare and the state of the NHS.

British Household Panel Survey

The British Household Panel Survey (BHPS) has been used to investigate:

- working life and stress
- household density and mental health
- health of single homeless people
- women's well-being at work
- psychiatric consequences of leaving home and relationship break-down.

This is by no means an exhaustive list of either useful sources or potential topics. Much research of interest remains to be done using the multiplicity of data available from the Archive and researchers are advised to seek assistance from DA staff in locating potential sources of information for their research topics.

Quality assurance

If researchers are to have confidence that the data supplied to them by the DA are suitable for use then the DA has a responsibility to ensure that the data it holds:

- have come from a reliable and reputable source
- are without obvious bias
- preserve appropriate confidentiality
- are provided within a proper legal framework – with both data owners and prospective data users signing legal agreements covering the terms and conditions for the dissemination and use of the data.

To fulfil these responsibilities the DA plays a crucial role in checking the content and provenance of data resources. This requires that full documentation that describes the data is obtained. The data producers are asked to provide comprehensive information on the:

- aims and objectives of the original project
- range of information collected
- methodology used for data collection – details of sampling and weighting, instruments (e.g. questionnaires) used, coding frames
- structure and content of dataset
- confidentiality or sensitivity of data

and a bibliography.

On receipt of a dataset the DA undertakes an evaluation and validation process to ensure its quality and usability. The dataset is checked for errors and inconsistency and then converted into standard formats (SPSS, Stata, SAS, etc.) for statistical analysis. The documentation is converted to a standard format for dissemination and a copy of both the data and documentation is held in the Archive. The DA works closely with the data producer during this process to resolve any queries or errors found. Workshops held by the DA offer feedback to data producers with a view to improving future resources. At the same time secondary users of data gain insight into potential effective and informed use of the resources.

Confidentiality constraints

Many of the data resources that are most useful for health research bring with them issues of sensitivity and confidentiality. If data are to be made available to the research community, it is essential to ensure that sensitive information and the confidentiality of the survey respondents are respected – be they individuals, households, institutions or organisations. Providers of administrative data must be confident that their information is not being misused. At the same time it is important that necessary safeguards do not reduce the usefulness of the data to an unacceptable extent. The DA has extensive experience in dealing with these issues and offers advice and support to data producers in order to achieve an acceptable balance between confidentiality and open access. A data user must guarantee to abide by the constraints of confidentiality required by the data source.

How to access the Data Archive

DA services

It is the role of the Archive to encourage and enable research. Its systems are designed to assist the researcher in identifying suitable material and obtaining speedy access to relevant data. The DA offers:

- a Web-searchable catalogue of holdings
- a dataset User Guide for every dataset
- experienced staff in the Archive User Services Section.

The DA Web pages (http://dawww.essex.ac.uk) contain a large amount of relevant information including:

- the DA catalogue with comprehensive indexing of a subject category listing, to enable users to locate material of interest
- full dataset documentation describing each study's data creation process, methodology and list of variables
- links to the Archive's Major Studies list, other archives and social science information services grouped by country.

There are several ways to search the Archive's data holdings for the data you need. Once in the Web pages, follow the Searching for Data link. From there you can do the following.

Search BIRON

Bibliographic Information Retrieval Online (BIRON) is the DA's primary search engine. Searches are performed on catalogue records (study descriptions) and keywords describing the studies in the Archive's collection. BIRON provides information on:

- the topics investigated
- where the research was carried out
- when the data were collected
- responsibility for the research/data collection
- Data Archive study numbers
- titles or part titles
- sampling procedures
- spatial units
- methods of data collection
- abstracts or research purposes.

Full study descriptions can be displayed on screen. These descriptions are usually sufficient to enable users to identify studies suitable to their purposes which can then be ordered from the Archive.

Search the 'Subject Categories' listing under 'Health'

Through this route users will be able to browse a list of datasets where health or health-related topics are the key component of the dataset.

Browse the list of 'Major Studies'

Users may also browse a title list of the major datasets held by the Archive by following the link to Major Studies.

Link to other sites and resources

This provides a comprehensive list of links to other archives and social science information services, grouped by country.

For many of the Archive's more popular datasets the contextual documentation which describes the data creation process and methodology is available to view on-line, as are fully labelled variable listings. These enable users to assess further whether a dataset is suitable for the intended purpose once they have identified likely resources using the BIRON search interface. Use the Archive Web pages and follow the Online documentation link to obtain more information. In addition, a full bibliography is provided with the description of each dataset held in BIRON and we suggest that

89

potential researchers consult this to gain an insight into the type and range of research that has been undertaken using these datasets. Help is available from the staff of the Data Archive to locate relevant sources and to refine BIRON searches.

Obtaining data from the DA

Data are available from the Archive in a variety of formats and on a variety of media. Having identified the dataset required either by using BIRON or contacting the Archive Users' Services Section, the researcher needs to:

- complete a data access application form. This can be downloaded in Word 6 format from the website or alternatively completed on-line
- sign the User Agreement form. In signing this form the user agrees to abide by conditions stipulated by the data producer with regard to the use of this specific data
- send the completed forms to:

The Data Archive	Tel:	01206 872001
User Services Section	Fax:	01206 872003
University of Essex	E-mail: archive@essex.ac.uk
Colchester	http://dawww.essex.ac.uk
Essex CO4 3SQ	

Future developments

Two central issues face users of datasets: first, identifying and locating relevant sources of information; second, assessing whether the resources are suitable for the intended purpose. The services provided by the DA are an excellent first step. However, much more can be achieved and the Archive plans to expand its services for users in two key areas by:

- establishing an 'information gateway' to health data, providing information on key resources wherever they are located
- provision of on-line browsing and simple analysis facilities for the data as well as the contextual documentation and lists of variables.

The mechanisms used will be both strategic and operational. The Archive is developing strategic partnerships and implementing flexible methods to provide access to important research resources.

These will enable it to access sources previously difficult to locate or perhaps held under restricted confidentiality conditions.

Steps to be taken include:

- negotiating full access to a dataset, where the Archive is itself the primary manager and supplier of the data
- where data is held and managed by others
  - negotiating data exchange agreements
  - providing an information resource about such data
  - brokering access for UK researchers; enabling access, for example, to commercially sensitive data.

Use of new technologies and systems developed through an EU-funded programme will also enable the Archive to provide information about, and access to, a wide range of data held all over the world. Though the NESSTAR system (Networked Social Science Tools and Resources) users will have a common interface on the Internet to the data holdings of a large number of worldwide providers and disseminators of statistical information. NESSTAR enables users to:

- locate multiple data sources across national boundaries
- browse detailed metadata about these data
- analyse and visualise the data on-line
- download subsets of data in one of a number of formats for local use.

The system will include advanced user authentication procedures to prevent unauthorised use of the data. The DA intends to use NESSTAR to hold all key empirical data on-line, including major health surveys, within an integrated gateway and search system providing easy access. The first edition of NESSTAR was made available to users in the spring of 2000 – an appropriate and exciting start to the new millennium.

7 National health surveys

Madhavi Bajekal

Introduction

National health surveys provide an important mechanism to collect comprehensive information on the health status of the population. Information about the health of the population demonstrates a familiar paradox: namely, the density of data available is inversely proportional to the well-known pyramid of ill-health, disease and mortality in the population at any given time. While mortality data are the most complete, these provide an objective measure of only one dimension of health. Data that record process statistics, such as hospital admission data, are often used as proxy measures of population morbidity. However, by their very nature, service utilisation data miss out the large proportion of symptoms and disease that are not reported to medical practitioners. This is true even in the UK where universal health coverage under the NHS and the 'gate-keeper' role of GPs limit distortions in utilisation and referral patterns found in fee-based or insurance-funded systems.

The defining attributes of national health surveys, which distinguish them from ad-hoc surveys, are that they are an ongoing series with a defined long-term programme. The structure and content of national health surveys carried out in various countries is guided crucially by the aims of the survey. All such surveys serve a public health monitoring function, which can usually be met by sampling a representative cross-section of the population. However, national health surveys which aim beyond monitoring to understand the causal determinants of health or the movement of people into and out of variable states of health require the inclusion of a panel or longitudinal element in the survey design.

In this chapter we focus on the Health Survey for England, set up in 1991, with the aims of monitoring the health of the population and progress towards defined *Health of the Nation* targets.

Background and aims of the HSE

The Health Survey for England (HSE) is a series of annual surveys commissioned by the Department of Health. The survey is designed to be representative of the general, non-institutional population living in England and provides a measure of the health status of the population. Since 1994, the Joint Health Surveys Unit comprising the National Centre for Social Research (formerly Social and Community Planning Research) and the Department of Epidemiology, University College, London have carried out the survey every year.

The survey aims to:

- provide annual data about the nation's health
- monitor key indicators of progress to support *Our Healthier Nation* strategy
- examine inequalities in health between population subgroups
- estimate the proportion of the population with specific health conditions and the prevalence of risk factors associated with those conditions.

A major strength of the HSE, which differentiates it from other general health surveys, is that the health questionnaire is followed by a nurse visit during which various physical measurements, tests and samples of blood and saliva are collected. These measurements constitute an integral part of the survey and provide biomedical information about known risk factors associated with disease (e.g. cholesterol level, blood pressure) as well as simple physiological measurements (e.g. lung function tests, waist–hip ratio). Biological markers also provide objective validation for self-reported behaviour, such as assays of serum and saliva cotinine, a metabolite of nicotine, used to cross-check reported smoking behaviour.

Survey design

The HSE was designed to provide data at both national and regional level about the population living in private households in England. The health surveys in the series to date have all adopted a similar multistage stratified probability sampling design. The first stage involves a systematic selection of 720 postcode sectors, or primary sampling units (PSU), comprising a 1 in 10 sample of all postcode sectors in England. Before selection, the list of postal sectors is stratified by health region and a range of other socio-economic factors to maximise the precision of the sample. In the second stage, a specified number of addresses (e.g. 21 in 1998) are systematically selected from each selected PSU using a residential address listing supplied by the Post Office (the small users Postcode Address File) as the sampling frame.

The 1991 and 1992 surveys had a limited population sample of about 3000 and 4000 adults, respectively. From 1993 onwards, the adult sample size was increased to about 16 000 to enable analysis by socio-economic characteristics and health regions. A sample of about 4000 children aged between 2 and 15 was introduced for the first time in 1995. From then onwards, total sample size has remained at about 20 000 comprising a general population cross-section of approximately 4 in 10 000 persons aged 2 and over.

In years where the survey focus is on special population groups (e.g. minority ethnic groups in 1999), the numbers in the sub-populations of interest are 'boosted' to provide a sample large enough for comparative subgroup analysis. To allow over-sampling in this way within the survey's annual budget, there is a concomitant reduction in the size of the general cross-section of population sampled in the year.

Interviewing on the HSE is conducted throughout the year to take account of seasonal differences. Response rates to the survey are consistently high (averaging about 78% between 1994 and 1998) and quality standards are maintained using highly trained interviewers and rigorous quality control checks on laboratory results. Interviews are conducted by computer-assisted methods.

Subject content

The HSE has evolved a rolling programme which retains continuity in key topics from year to year as well as allowing flexibility in detailed coverage of specific disease areas or population subgroups (*see* Table 7.1). The criteria for inclusion of a topic in the 'core' repeated every year are that it:

- measures a target (e.g. former *Health of the Nation* targets such as obesity, blood pressure[1,2]) or is an indicator of progress towards health targets

95

Table 7.1: Programme of the HSE 1993/99

	HSE93	HSE94	HSE95	HSE96	HSE97	HSE98	HSE99
Sample Size							
Adults (16+)	16539	15809	16055	16443	8582	15908	c. 13500
Children (2–15)			3733	3885	6964	3746	c. 4500
Core Topics							
Self-reported							
General health	●	●	●	●	●	●	●
Smoking	●	●	●	●	●	●	●
Drinking	●	●	●	●	●	●	●
Psychosocial health (GHQ12)	●	●	●		●		
Socio-economic status (e.g. social class/ethnicity/ education/employment/ income/tenure)	●	●	●	●	●	●	●
Use of health services	●	●	●	●	●	●	●
Birth weight of children			●	●	●	●	●
Measurements & medicines							
Body mass index (BMI) (height(m^2)/weight (kg))	●	●	●	●	●	●	●
Blood pressure	●	●	●	●	●	●	●
Haemoglobin/ferritin	●	●		●	●	●	●
Cotinine (saliva/serum)	●	●		●	●	●	●
Nicotine replacement		●		●	●	●	●
Prescribed medicines	●	●	●	●	●	●	●
Contraceptive pill/HRT 98,99	●	●	●	●	●	●	●
Vitamin supplements	●	●	●	●	●	●	●
Disease-specific Focus							
CVD conditions and risk factors							
Chest pain, diagnosed CVD conditions and diabetes	●	●				●	●
Social support	●	●	●			●	●
Parental history of CVD	●	●				●	●
Variety/control at work	●	●					
Stress	●	●					
Waist–hip ratio	●	●			●	●	●
Blood – cholesterol	●	●				●	●
Blood – fibrinogen	●	●				●	●
Glycosylated haemoglobin	●	●					●
Blood – C reactive protein						●	●
Blood – fasting glucose (35+)					●		
Blood – triglycerides (35+)					●		
ECG (35+)							●
Respiratory/atopic conditions							
MRC respiratory questionnaire	●	●	●	●		●	●
Asthma			●	●	●		●
Hay fever, eczema			●	●			
Indoor pollutants/allergens			●				
Lung function			●	●	●		●
Blood – IgE/HDM IgE			●	●	●		●
Physical activity/exercise	●	●			●	●	●
Eating habits	●	●			●	●	●
Disability			●				
Accidents			●	●	●		●
Health status (Euroqol/SF36)				●			
Strengths and difficulties (4–15)					●		●
Population Focus							
General, non-institutional	●	●	●	●	●	●	●
Young people					●		
Minority ethnic groups							●

- is required to interpret other data such as an underlying risk factor for many diseases (e.g. smoking, drinking)
- is a cross-sectional variable by which other factors would need to be analysed (e.g. indicators of socio-economic status)
- measures the impact of the disease on healthcare utilisation (e.g. GP consultations, medication, hospital services).

In recognition of the broader social determinants of health, multiple measures of individual socio-economic status (such as employment status, social class, car ownership, tenure, level of education, family composition and income), and ethnic origin are asked in every cycle of the health survey.

In addition to the core topics, each year the survey focuses on one or more health conditions that are revisited periodically to assess change over time. This introduces an important element of dynamic adaptability in the coverage of the HSE to reflect emerging health concerns and priorities. The first four years of the survey (1991/94) concentrated on cardiovascular disease and associated risk factors. Since 1995, the survey has investigated a wide range of conditions such as respiratory illnesses, allergies, non-fatal accidents and dis-abilities. In response to the new policy initiatives outlined in the consultative document *Our Healthier Nation*,[3] the HSE in 2000 will focus on social exclusion and the health of elderly people living in the community and in institutional care.

Specific modules are included in the HSE if they meet all or most of the criteria listed below.

- The information needed reflects public health objectives and priorities.
- The prevalence of the disease/condition is such that a sample size of approximately 20 000 or less would provide representative responses for age, sex and socio-economic groups.
- The information is currently not available from other sources or it is proposed that the health survey replace those sources.
- The information is amenable to collection from a community-based survey, i.e. the questions would be acceptable to respondents.

Context and linkages

The HSE is part of an overall survey programme, which includes the National Psychiatric Morbidity Survey of the Department of Health, and the National Diet and Nutrition Surveys of the Department of Health and the Ministry of Agriculture, Fisheries and Food. These specialist surveys cover the more detailed information needs in the areas of mental health and nutrition. However, the HSE collects more general indicators of nutritional status (e.g. haemoglobin levels, food frequency questionnaire) and psychological well-being as measured by the General Health Questionnaire (GHQ12).[4]

From 1994 onwards, permission has been sought from respondents on the health survey to 'flag' their records on the National Health Service Central Register (NHSCR). This will allow cause of death information to be added to the survey data at a future date making it possible to link individual behaviour, lifestyle and morbidity with cause of death.

Accessing the HSE data

The HSE data for each year are deposited in the ESRC Data Archive in the form of portable SPSS data files (*see* Chapter 6 for a more detailed description of the work of the Archive, and how to access data held there). To protect data confidentiality, personal details other than age, sex and health authority of residence are not included on the dataset. Besides the household and individual level variables collected as part of the survey, the datasets also include all derived variables (e.g. body mass index, equivalised household income) used in the analyses presented in the annual reports. This ensures consistency in definitions of variables between users and across different years of the survey. To ensure that sample design effects due to clustering and non–response bias are properly taken into account in the calculation of standard errors, weighting factors for key variables are included in the public access datasets.

In addition to the comprehensive and detailed coverage of survey results provided in the annual HSE reports,[5–11] specially commissioned ad-hoc analyses and reference tables have recently been released in electronic form.[12,13] These can be accessed either on the Department of Health website (http:/www. doh.gov.uk/public) or on CD-ROM on request from the Department of Health.

The full set of questions for the Health Survey for England

1991/96 is held in the Question Bank at the Centre for Applied Social Surveys, which is an ESRC resource centre run jointly by the National Centre for Social Research and the Universities of Southampton and Surrey.[14] As far as possible, questions on the HSE conform to the set of harmonised questions common across surveys and the national census in order to enhance comparability of information from different sources.

Complementary sources

In addition to the Health Survey for England, the Health Education Authority commissions a number of nationally representative ad-hoc surveys, primarily focussing on health promotion and health education. The Health Education Authority has compiled a comparative overview of over 40 major health and lifestyle surveys in the UK conducted between 1989 and 1996.[15] The database is available on CD-ROM and can be searched either by topic, which are categorised by key *Health of the Nation* target areas, or by selecting specific surveys. The information on each survey covers sample sizes, survey frequency, full text of the questionnaire, publication details and, where available, summary results.

Use of the HSE data in analysis: an illustrative example

The range and depth of coverage of the HSE provides a valuable source of population morbidity data to suit a variety of analyses. The data are available in a format that allows a range of analyses suitable for research, planning or policy concerns. Listed below are potential types of analyses that are possible using the HSE data.

- Investigating patterns and trends in the prevalence of disease and associated risk factors at the national level over time.
- Providing estimates of self-reported morbidity – annually at broad regional levels and, by aggregating data over a number of years, for smaller localities such as health authorities.
- Measuring inequalities in health and disease between population subgroups by socio-economic status, ethnicity, household income levels, and neighbourhood deprivation.
- Epidemiological analyses, e.g. exploring the relationship between individual risk factors, personal disadvantage and area level

deprivation and the interactions between them to understand better the contribution of compositional and contextual elements of health inequalities.

- Health services research, e.g. quantification of health services utilisation in relation to individual morbidity and socio-economic indicators.

In response to the increasing emphasis on local priorities and local targets in the health strategy outlined in the government's consultative Green Paper, *Our Healthier Nation*, now issued as *Saving Lives: our healthier nation*, HSE data were used to produce estimates of morbidity at the level of health authorities (HAs) for the first time.[11] Key considerations in using retrospective HSE data to calculate local morbidity measures were the adequacy of the sample size, the representativeness of the sample in terms of population and geographical coverage, the selection of candidate variables and the method of standardisation and reporting to allow local areas to compare their estimates to similar types of areas and with national rates.

It was clear from the outset that the HSE sample size of 16 000 adults in each year was too small at HA level to allow the calculation of robust estimates which took into account the key correlates of health, namely age and gender. It was decided to combine data over the three years 1994/96, as these were the most recent years for which data were available and were also years when a straightforward cross-section of the population was selected (unlike the following year, 1997, when the sample of young persons under 25 was 'boosted'). The HSE records for these three years were then linked to current (1998) health authority boundaries using the postcode of the survey respondent to identify their current HA of residence on the centrally maintained postcode-to-HA look-up file.

Pooling data over the three years yielded on average 500 counts per health authority (range 148–1046), with an approximate 50:30:20 split between young (16–44), middle-aged (45–64) and older (65+) age ranges and just over 54% female. On comparing the sample counts with the mid-1996 population estimates for HAs, the age/sex distribution in the two datasets was found to be broadly similar and sample size per HA highly correlated with HA population size (0.9, p=0.001). In other words, the fraction of the total population sampled (mean 12.5 per 10 000) was consistent across areas, with smaller counts in less populated HAs and vice versa.

As noted above, the HSE contains a core set of topics that are repeated every year and which could therefore be combined across years. From this core set, 22 health indicators were identified (Box 7.1) which highlight differences between HA populations in:

- levels of morbidity as measured by self-assessed general health and rates of chronic and acute illness
- the prevalence of risk factors such as obesity, high blood pressure, excess alcohol consumption and smoking, and
- respiratory conditions such as asthma and wheeze; psychosocial health as measured by the GHQ12; and accident rates.

Box 7.1: Morbidity indicators available at health authority level

General health, chronic and acute illness
Proportion with self-assessed fair, bad, or very bad health
Prevalence of longstanding illness
Prevalence of acute sickness
Proportion of adults on prescribed medication

Blood pressure
Mean systolic blood pressure
Mean diastolic blood pressure
Proportion with high blood pressure

Body Mass Index and obesity
Mean height of adults (cm)
Mean weight of adults (kg)
Mean Body Mass Index (BMI) of adults
Proportion of adults who are overweight
Proportion of adults who are obese

Smoking and drinking
Proportion of adults who currently smoke cigarettes, pipes or cigars
Proportion of adults who currently smoke cigarettes
Proportion of adults with a serum cotinine level of 20 ng/ml or over
Mean per capita number of cigarettes smoked
Proportion of males drinking over 21 units/week and females drinking over 14 units/week
Proportion of males drinking over 50 units/week and females drinking over 35 units/week
Mean weekly alcohol consumption (base all adults)

Respiratory illness
Proportion with wheeze or doctor-diagnosed asthma

Psychiatric morbidity
Proportion of adults with GHQ12 score of 4 and over
Major accident rates
Annual accident rate per 100 persons for major accidents

Source: Health Survey for England 1994–1996.[12]

For each of the 22 indicators separate prevalence estimates were calculated for men, women and persons. In order to compare estimates between HAs, the overall prevalence estimates were age standardised to the European reference population. Given the relatively small base sample at HA level, the counts were split into three age breaks – the young (16–44), middle-aged (45–64) and retired (65+) – rather than the usual 10-year age groups, to calculate age-specific rates for each HA. These were used to calculate the overall standardised rate using the method of direct standardisation. The tables also contain the 95% confidence limits for both the crude and standardised values after taking into account complex survey design effects due to clustering.[6] The reference population and the method of standardisation is similar to that used for the mortality-based indicators at HA level included in the Public Health Common Database,[16] thereby facilitating comparisons between the indices of morbidity and mortality at the local level. Furthermore, each table contains reference rates for England as a whole, as well as averages for six area clusters [17] to allow HAs to compare their results nationally as well as with similar types of areas.

Figure 7.1 shows the range of variation in the standardised proportion of persons rating their health as either 'fair', 'poor' or 'bad' on a five-point scale. Given the small sample size by HA, the 95% confidence intervals are wide. Nevertheless, 18 HAs show rates that are significantly higher than the England average while 18 are significantly lower than average. There is 2.5-fold variation (95% CI; 1.7–3.9) in self-assessed health between the HA with the highest and lowest rates which is considerably higher than the corresponding ratio in age-standardised all-cause mortality rates of 1.5 over the same period 1994/96.[16] Poor self-assessed health and all-cause mortality rates at HA level are highly correlated ($r=0.74$, *see* Figure 7.2), but urban areas such as Manchester and Liverpool are notable outliers where self-assessed health appears to be much better than expected, given their high mortality rates. When patterns are examined by type of areas as characterised by ONS clusters, both types of data show relatively poorer health in Inner London and mining and industrial areas and good health in rural and prospering areas. These data support the growing literature which show that self-assessed health status may be the best predictor of current and future morbidity, disability and premature mortality.

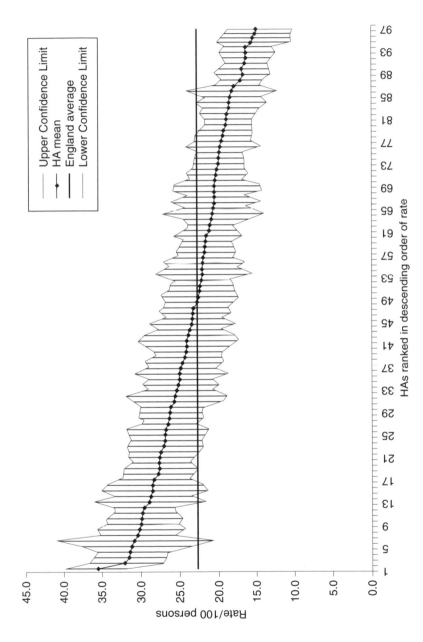

Figure 7.1 Variation in self-assessed poor health by HA. *Source*: Health Survey for England 1994–1996.[12]

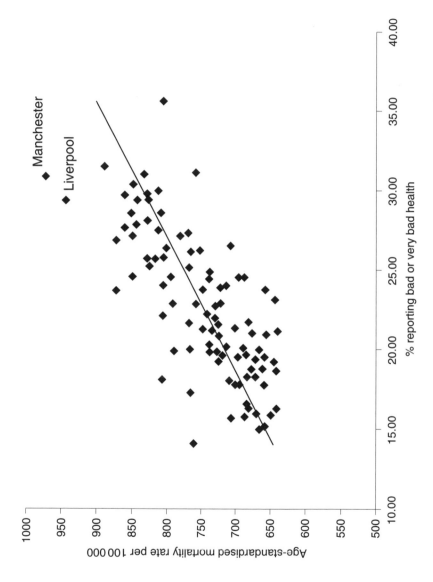

Figure 7.2 Poor health vs mortality rate. *Source:* Health Survey for England 1994–1996.[12]

Conclusion

The above analysis provides one example of the potential of the HSE data to advance our understanding of the contribution of underlying social, contextual and behavioural factors in explaining inequalities in health. With the survey currently in its tenth year, the range and depth of information collected makes it an invaluable resource for research, healthcare planning and policy formulation.

References

1   Department of Health (1991) *Health of the Nation: a consultative document for Health in England.* Cmd 1523. HMSO, London.

2   Department of Health (1992) *Health of the Nation: a strategy for health in England.* Cmd 1986. HMSO, London.

3   Department of Health (1998) *Our Healthier Nation: a contract for health.* Cmd 3852. The Stationery Office, London.

4   Goldberg DP, Williams P (1988) *A User's Guide to the General Health Questionnaire.* NFER-Nelson, Windsor.

5   Prescott-Clarke P and Primatesta P (eds) (1998) *Health Survey for England: the health of young people '95–97. Vols1 & 2.* HMSO, London.

6   Prescott-Clarke P and Primatesta P (eds) (1998) *Health Survey for England 1996. Vols1 & 2.* HMSO, London.

7   Prescott-Clarke P and Primatesta P (eds) (1997) *Health Survey for England 1995. Vols1 & 2.* HMSO, London.

8   Colhoun H and Prescott-Clarke P (eds) (1996) *Health Survey for England 1994. Vols1 & 2.* HMSO, London.

9   Bennett N *et al.* (1995) *Health Survey for England 1993.* HMSO, London.

10 Breeze E *et al.* (1994) *Health Survey for England 1992.* HMSO, London.

11 White A *et al.* (1993) *Health Survey for England 1991.* HMSO, London.

12 Bajekal M (1999) *Health Survey for England: geographical variation in health indicators by health authority, 1994–1996.* CD-ROM, 1999. Produced by Social and Community Planning Research. Contact Michelle Marcelle, Department of Health, Skipton House, 80 London Road, London SE1 6LW, for a copy of the tables on a CD-ROM. Also available at http://www.doh.gov.uk/public.

13 Social and Community Planning Research (1999) *Health Survey for England: adults reference tables, 1997.* Available at http://www.doh.gov.uk/public.

14   Centre for Applied Social Surveys. *Question Bank*. National Centre for Social Research, University of Southampton, and University of Surrey. E-mail: cassqb@natcen.ac.uk.

15   Health Education Authority (1996) *Health and Lifestyles*. National Surveys Guide CD-ROM, version 1.

16   Department of Health (1997) *Public Health Common Dataset 1997*. CD-ROM. Produced by the National Institute of Epidemiology, University of Surrey.

17   Wallace M and Denham C (1996) *ONS Classification of Local and Health Authorities of Great Britain*. Studies on Medical and Population Studies No. 59. HMSO, London.

8 Assessment of clinical and health outcomes within the National Health Service in England

Azim Lakhani

Introduction

This chapter is based on the work of the National Centre for Health Outcomes Development in England. It shows how official statistics have been used to address key questions concerning health outcomes and the contribution of healthcare to such outcomes in England. It also shows the limitations of the use of official statistics and how they may be supplemented locally with special data collection.

The following quote in the National Health Service (NHS) Executive's publication *A Guide to the National Health Service*[1] articulates the health outcomes goals of the NHS:

> The fundamental purpose of the NHS is to secure through the resources available the greatest possible improvement in the physical and mental health of the people of England by promoting health, preventing ill-health, diagnosing and treating injury and disease and caring for those with long-term illness and disability who require the services of the NHS.
>
> Sir Alan Langlands, Chief Executive

Specific health outcomes questions facing the NHS

A First Class Service

The government consultation document, *A First Class Service*,[2] set out three aspects of a strategy to drive the improvement of performance in the NHS by:

- setting clear standards
- delivering standards by promoting effective delivery of high quality services locally, and
- monitoring standards by ensuring that there are strong monitoring mechanisms in place externally.

NHS Performance Assessment Framework

Performance assessment is central to all these activities. *A First Class Service* highlighted the need for a performance framework which would support the drive for higher quality standards, ensuring that performance assessment is focused on the delivery of clinically and cost-effective, appropriate and timely health services to meet local needs. A document entitled *The NHS Performance Assessment Framework*,[3] published following a consultation exercise, describes the following six areas of performance.

1 **Health improvement** – to reflect the over-arching aims of improving the general health of the population and of reducing health inequalities, which are influenced by many factors, reaching well beyond the NHS.
2 **Fair access** - to recognise that the NHS' contribution must begin by offering fair access to its services in relation to people's needs, irrespective of geography, socio-economic group, ethnicity, age or sex.
3 **Effective delivery of appropriate healthcare** - to recognise that fair access must be to care that is effective, appropriate and timely, and complies with agreed standards.
4 **Efficiency** – to ensure that the effective care is delivered with a minimum of waste, and that the NHS uses its resources to achieve value for money.
5 **Patient and carer experience** – to assess the way in which patients and their carers experience and view the quality of the care they receive, to ensure that the NHS is sensitive to individual needs.
6 **Health outcomes of the NHS care** – to assess the direct contribution of the NHS care to improvements in overall health, and complete the circle back to the over-arching goal of health improvement.

Each of the six areas may be divided further into more specific aspects of performance. For example, health outcomes of NHS care is described as NHS success in using its resources to:

- reduce levels of risk factors
- reduce levels of diseases and impairment
- reduce complications of treatment
- improve quality of life for patients and carers
- reduce premature death.

Official statistics may be harnessed to monitor achievement in relation to standards set for each of the six areas of the performance framework. This may be achieved through the production of comparative data at national level or measurement at local level. This chapter will show how this has been attempted within the NHS in England over a number of years in the context of two of the performance assessment areas, i.e. health improvement and health outcomes of the NHS care.

The National Centre for Health Outcomes Development

The National Centre for Health Outcomes Development (NCHOD) is a key source of information on assessment of levels of health and outcomes of health interventions, at individual, health authority, NHS hospital trust and local authority levels for the English NHS and the government. It is based jointly at the London School of Hygiene and Tropical Medicine, University of London and the Institute of Health Sciences, University of Oxford. In 1993, the Department of Health in England set up the Central Health Outcomes Unit (CHOU) to coordinate a programme of work to develop methods and systems necessary to assess health outcomes. Following the evolution of a substantial national programme, the unit was contracted out in 1998 and became what is now the NCHOD.

Over the years the CHOU and the NCHOD have commissioned and developed a variety of sets of comparative data, for example the Public Health Common Data Set, Population Health Outcome Indicators, Clinical Indicators and Cancer Survival Indicators, among others. These are based predominantly on analyses of routinely available data undertaken for the NCHOD by institutions such as the Centre for Public Health Monitoring at the London

School of Hygiene and Tropical Medicine. The indicators have now been brought together within a *Clinical and Health Outcomes Knowledge Base,* alongside other relevant information, by the NCHOD.[4]

Challenges in harnessing official statistics to address such questions

Any serious attempt at addressing the kinds of questions listed within the health improvement and outcomes sections of the performance framework poses a number of challenges relating to:

• concepts

• technical issues

• uses and usefulness of data.

Each of these is discussed in more detail below.

Challenges relating to concepts

Definitions

The first challenge relates to varying definitions and levels of understanding of the term 'outcome'. Some people regard 'outcome' as a state of health or well-being at a point in time. Others regard it as a change in state. However, for some patients, for example those with physical disability, there may not be much change in the level of disability from one point in time to another. This may still be considered an outcome, even a positive outcome as the alternative might have been a deterioration in the level of disability. Yet others consider outcome as a result (an attributable effect). This requires measurement not just of the health state or change but also attribution of that state to an intervention, and as a result can only be expressed as a result of something and not as a result in isolation. Yet others define outcome as a benefit, given that the objectives of the NHS are to offer a variety of benefits as described by the performance assessment framework. Hence success should be measured in terms of the benefit actually achieved. It is important to have common understanding and agreement of definitions as this will influence the way in which statistics are harnessed.

Types of outcomes

There are different kinds of outcomes, such as health outcomes and other outcomes, e.g. economic. The type of outcome being measured does need to be specified. If it is to be measured in terms of 'health' then this raises a new set of issues. For example, ill health may be measured in terms of:

- a biological state, e.g. biochemical changes in the blood
- physical impairment, e.g. blindness
- clinical signs and symptoms, e.g. swelling or tenderness
- function, e.g. mobility
- feeling of well-being, or
- impact on quality of life.

Outcomes as results

If outcome is described as a result then it may be important to state what it is a result of. This creates its own difficulties. For example, a state of health may be a result of the health service offering a treatment or alternatively, a result of the health service either not intervening at all or not intervening on time. Examples include prevention and treatment of acute asthma attacks as shown in Figure 8.1.[4] This figure also shows how a particular health state may be the collective result of the natural history of a health problem and the results of healthcare and wider efforts of society. Attribution may thus be very complicated. In some cases there may be little that the health services can do and a particular health end-point may be inevitable. Thus when an outcome is meant to reflect a result, it is very important to understand the extent to which that particular state of health is amenable to change. Health outcomes as results should be measured in the context of specific health outcome objectives, based on an understanding, from scientific evaluation of interventions, of the extent to which such change may be possible. The Central Health Outcomes Unit defined health outcome as an attributable effect of intervention or its lack on a previous health state.[5]

Perspectives

In choosing which outcome to measure there may be a number of perspectives which may vary. For example, in considering outcomes among patients with asthma, doctors may be concerned about levels of lung function while patients may be more concerned about whether they are able to sleep at night. Perspectives may vary

Health outcomes

Potential interventions

Proactive interventions
to avoid risk

Health professionals work with patients and their families to help avoid known causes, e.g. house dust mites. Comparative routine data on NHS activity and the cost of such activity to the NHS and wider society are not available at national level.

Exposure to amenable determinants
of asthma and acute attacks

There is uncertainty about some of the causes of asthma and acute attacks, i.e. some allergens, maternal smoking, air pollutants, dietary sodium, psychosocial problems, viral infection etc. There is a need for more research on causes. Comparative routine data on incidence and prevalence of causes are not available at national level.

Reactive interventions
to reduce risk

Comparative routine data about health professional activity on risk reduction, rates of prescription of prophylactic pharmaceutical drugs and balance between prevention and treatment are not available at national level.

Incidence
of asthma and acute attacks

There is lack of agreement on criteria for the diagnosis of asthma. Prevalence figures in the research literature range from 3–4% (all ages) and 5–15% (children). Comparative routine data on incidence and prevalence of asthma are not readily available at national level.

Timely interventions
to detect and treat asthma

Health professionals work with patients, their families and schools to enhance self care, e.g. use of peak flow meters, timely use of pharmaceutical drugs etc. Estimated 1992/3 direct NHS expenditure on, e.g. GP consultations, pharmaceutical treatment, outpatients attendance etc. was £400m (*Source:* DoH, *Burdens of Disease*, 1996). Comparative routine data on these are not available at national level.

Potentially avoidable adverse consequences –
severity, secondary disease and complications of treatment

Confidential enquiries suggest that some of the prolonged and severe attacks of asthma and their complications are potentially avoidable. Comparative routine data on the incidence of increased severity/complications are not available at national level.

Late interventions
to minimise consequences

Estimated 1992/3 direct NHS expenditure on hospitalisation was £40m (*Source:* DoH, *Burdens of Disease*, 1996). There is variation in hospitalisation rates. Confidential enquiries suggest that some acute episodes leading to hospitalisation are potentially avoidable.

Impact on function and quality of life

A local audit (*BMJ* 1992; **304**:361–4) showed 51% of asthma patients waking up at night with wheeze; 45% wheezy at least once a week; 31% missed school or work in previous year; and 23% avoided certain physical activities. Comparative routine data on impact on quality of life and costs to society due to, e.g. time off work are not available at national level.

Premature death

There is geographical variation in death rates. Confidential enquiries suggest that some deaths are potentially avoidable (McColl *et al*; *Population Health Outcomes Indicators*, 1993)

Figure 8.1 Case study: asthma activity, resource use and outcomes. Crown copyright material from the NCHOD's Clinical and Health Outcomes Knowledge Base, reproduced with the permission of the Controller of Her Majesty's Stationery Office.

between clinicians, patients, carers, public health specialists, commissioners of healthcare, providers of healthcare, service managers, policymakers, the public, researchers and others.

All of the above have implications for measurement and the use of official statistics.

Challenges relating to the technical issues

Timing: short, medium and long-term outcomes

In some cases an outcome may manifest itself soon after a treatment, e.g. less pain after taking pain relief drugs. In other cases it may take many years, e.g. blindness as a complication of untreated diabetes. In the latter case it may become necessary to use proxy measures for outcome and measures of intermediate states. For example, if there is good scientific evidence that control of blood sugar with insulin in patients with diabetes is likely to prevent complications, then the level of appropriate treatment could be measured and act as a proxy, in anticipation of benefit in the future. Alternatively, an intermediate change in the state may be used, for example, the control of blood sugar level, which may itself indicate a lower chance of developing complications in the future.

Period of measurement

Outcome measurements may be presented as values at one point in time; across a period, e.g. a year; as a series of cross-sectional values showing trends over years; or as longitudinal measures, examining what happens to an individual patient or a group of patients over time.

Attribution

This may be very complicated. In many cases a particular state of health is a cumulative end-point of a whole range of services and interventions. For example, a heart attack or death following a heart attack could be the result of political decisions, environmental issues, patient behaviour, preventive health interventions, primary healthcare, diagnostic services, treatment, emergency care, etc. While heart attacks and death may be measured and reflected in official statistics, attributing them statistically to their respective causes is extremely difficult and is usually left to judgement based on prevailing circumstances. The context and the natural progression of a particular disease may need to be taken into account.

Completeness and quality of routine data

In interpreting outcomes data based on routine statistics, the completeness and quality of the data need to be taken into account. For example, if operations or diagnoses are not coded well in hospital records, then indicators which rely on such codes may show fewer events based on them and would be incomplete.

Explaining variation in comparative data

In looking at variation between institutions it is very important to ensure that the numerators and denominators used to analyse the indicator match between organisations as far as is possible. For example, differences between populations in deaths from certain diseases may reflect the level of such diseases in the populations and not necessarily the outcomes of treatment. Similarly, deaths or other adverse events in hospitals may reflect the types of illnesses, the severity of disease and the presence of concurrent illnesses among patients treated and not necessarily the outcome of treatment. In addition, some of the variation between organisations may be due to chance events which may vary between organisations and from year to year.

Challenges relating to uses and the usefulness of data

Types of uses

Indicators based on routine data may have a variety of uses, for example, policy-making, service planning, risk and performance management, service evaluation, resource allocation, research, informed choice of services made by service users, judging user satisfaction, professional education and development.

Service coverage by the indicators

There are issues concerning the extent to which the different services provided by the health services are covered by the indicators. For example, a small select set of indicators may be manageable but may reduce choice and distort priorities. Single indicators examined in isolation may also provide an incomplete picture.

Public use

The major challenge with producing indicators for public use is to ensure that they are technically correct as far as is possible and yet simple enough to be understood by the public.

Central vs local analyses

Central development of indicators ensures that there is standardisation of definitions, numerators and denominators, and hence comparability. However, this may reduce choice and flexibility and ownership by those who might end up using the indicators locally. Central production is also dependent on central collation and availability of the data and thus, on the speed of the slowest contributor. For example, cancer registration data in England are currently many years out of date. This also has implications for the timeliness of the publication of indicators and their potential usefulness.

Level of aggregation

There are issues concerning the unit of aggregation within indicators and the numbers making up the indicator values. Meaningful variation may only be detected when numbers are large and hence require analyses at a high level of aggregation, e.g. whole hospitals or health authorities with large populations. These may, however, mask variations within such organisations and may be too crude for meaningful comparison. Such aggregations may also be too broad for meaningful application at local level although they may show trends which are important and useful at national level. Smaller levels of aggregation, on the other hand, may lead to numbers which are too small for meaningful comparison, with the added risk of identifying individual clinicians and patients.

Follow-up work

Publication of the indicators on its own may have little impact. The role of such indicators in performance management needs to be considered, including the incentives for their use, the sanctions available and the levers for change.

Approaches to addressing such challenges

Much of the CHOU's and now the NCHOD's development work over the years has involved making the best possible use of existing information while developing better information and tools for the future, addressing some of the challenges described above. The NCHOD has now brought all the information arising from the development work together into a new website, the *Clinical and*

Health Outcomes Knowledge Base.[4] This is available to the NHS via an intranet, the NHSnet.

The Clinical and Health Outcomes Knowledge Base

This contains:

- a range of indicators with attached data tables, maps and graphs showing comparative values where available. New indicators and data will be added periodically as they are developed

- health outcome models showing the relationship between health outcomes, health interventions and resource use for a number of clinical areas, e.g. stroke, asthma, with indicators in the *Knowledge Base* mapped on to the models

- information on the relationship between the indicators and the NHS Performance Assessment Framework

- reports of studies undertaken to develop and evaluate indicators

- reports of case studies undertaken to follow up and investigate indicator findings

- reports on statistical and other methods used as part of health outcomes assessment

- reference to new sections being developed on outcome measurement instruments and outcomes projects undertaken elsewhere, plus links for the purposes of networking.

In 1995 the CHOU consulted the NHS on proposals for rationalising existing datasets and presenting the indicators in relation to health outcome models of the kind in Figure 8.2. Following a positive response, indicators in the *Knowledge Base* are now grouped by health conditions or topics and also mapped onto health outcome models. Table 8.1 is an example of the ways in which indicators may be grouped for one condition – cervical cancer. It shows the range of indicators available in the *Knowledge Base* and elsewhere, based on existing routine data as well as variants of individual indicators by type of analyses, age, gender, organisation and years for which data are available.

Examples of assessment of outcomes based on routinely collected data

The following indicators have been selected to illustrate how judgements about outcomes may be made based on them as well as how some of the constraints described above have been overcome.

Population-based analyses of mortality

A large proportion of the indicators in the *Knowledge Base* cover death as an outcome, given the availability of data on registered deaths, provided by the Office for National Statistics (ONS). Death certificates have a geographical marker based on the postal code of the place of residence of the deceased. It is thus possible to associate the deaths with NHS health authorities and use data on resident populations to calculate population-based death rates. Figure 8.2[6] shows directly age and sex-standardised death rates from all circulatory diseases among people under 75 years of age, resident in 100 health authorities in England, with data pooled for three years. The health authorities have been grouped on the basis of a classification of areas developed by the ONS. This enables the comparison of death rates between populations with similar social and demographic characteristics. There is significant variation in death rates, both between as well as within 'like' health authorities. The deaths reflect a cumulative end-point of a variety of influences and interventions as explained earlier.

Hospital-based analyses of mortality

Data from the records of patients treated within hospitals in the NHS in England are collated nationally as part of a system called Hospital Episode Statistics (HES). This is discussed in more detail in Chapter 4. Each hospital record has data on method of admission, diagnoses, operative procedures and the method of discharge (including death) among others. The unit of data collection is an 'episode' – relating to care under one consultant medical professional. Figure 8.3[7] shows data comparing NHS hospital trusts in England on directly age-standardised rates of deaths in hospital within 30 days of an operative procedure, following an emergency admission.

All episodes for individual patients within one continuous in-patient spell, including episodes following transfer to another hospital, have been linked using a matching technique based on

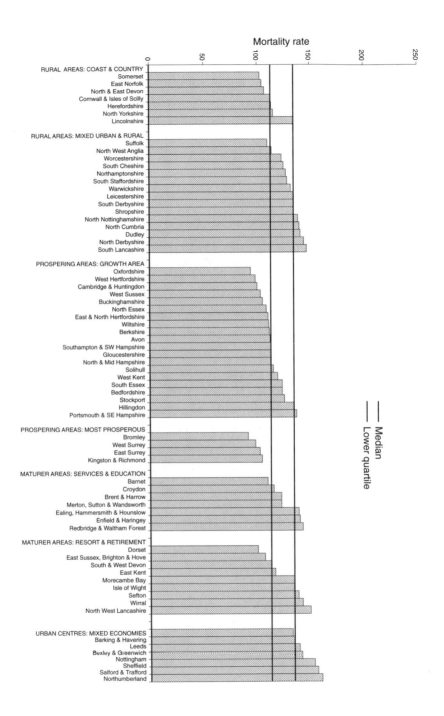

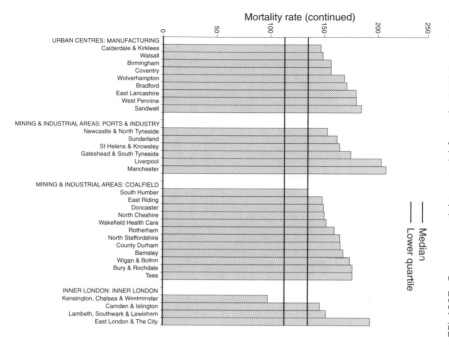

Figure 8.2 Deaths from all circulatory diseases (people under 75) 1997. Crown copyright material from the NHS Executive's High Level Performance Indicators, reproduced with the permission of the Controller of Her Majesty's Stationery Office.

Table 8.1: Indicators relating to cervical cancer

Indicator	Statistic	Sex*	Age group (variable)	Organisation**	Period (Year) Trend data	Current data
Screening for cervical cancer	Coverage: per cent of target population screened less than 5 years since last test	F	25–64	E, HA	89–99	99
Incidence based on registrations for cervical cancer	Indirectly age-standardised registration ratios (SRRs) and numbers of registrations	F	All ages	E&W, E, RO, GOR, ONS area, HA, LA	84–92	90–92
Incidence based on registrations for cervical cancer	Directly age-standardised registration rates and numbers of registrations	F	All ages	E&W, E, RO, GOR, ONS area, HA, LA	84–92	90–92
Mortality	Number of deaths	F	1+,1–4,5–14,15–34, 35–64,65–74,75+	E&W, E, RO, GOR, ONS area, HA, LA		97
Mortality	Average age-specific death rates	F	1+,1–4,5–14,15–34, 35–64,65–74,75+	E&W, E, RO, GOR, ONS area, HA, LA		95–97
Mortality	Indirectly standardised ratio (SMR)	F	All ages,15–64	E&W, E, RO, GOR, ONS area, HA, LA	88–97	95–97
Mortality	Directly standardised rate	F	15–64,65–74	E&W, E, RO, GOR, ONS area, HA, LA		95–97
Mortality	Years of life lost (number and rates)	F	Up to 75	E&W, E, RO, GOR, ONS area, HA, LA		95–97
Survival after diagnosis of cancer	1-year and 5-year relative survival (%)	F	15–99	E, RO, HA		89–90

*M, male; F, female; P, persons.
**England and Wales (E&W), England (E), NHS Executive Regional Office (RO), Standard Government Office Region (GOR), Office for National Statistics Area Classification (ONS area), Health Authority (HA), Local Authority (LA), Provider Unit (PU)

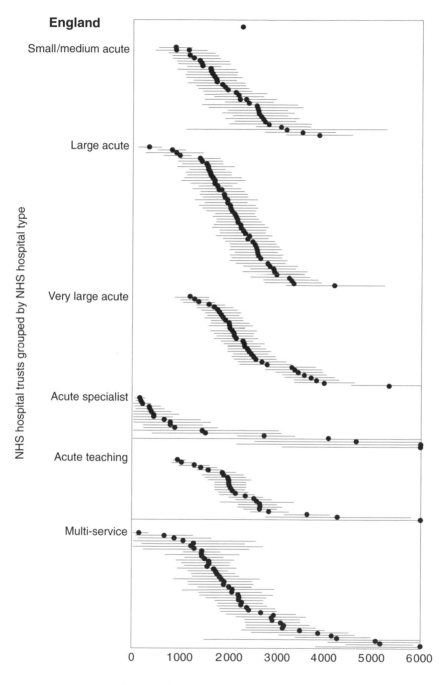

England

NHS hospital trusts grouped by NHS hospital type

Small/medium acute

Large acute

Very large acute

Acute specialist

Acute teaching

Multi-service

0   1000   2000   3000   4000   5000   6000

Age-standardised rate per 10000 and 95% confidence interval

Figure 8.3 Deaths in hospital within 30 days of surgery (all ages) by NHS hospital trust, grouped by hospital type (national summary), emergency admissions, England 1997–98. Crown copyright material from the NHS Executive's Clinical Indicators, reproduced with the permission of the Controller of Her Majesty's Stationery Office.

age, sex and postcode. A continuous inpatient spell (CIP) is defined as a continuous period of inpatient care within the NHS. It may include transfer from one hospital to another, even a hospital in another district. In the absence of names of patients or a unique identification number, episodes with a matching postal code, date of birth and sex are assumed to relate to the same patient. Such episodes are placed in chronological order. Decisions about whether sequential episodes are part of a CIP are made on the basis of information on episode order, discharge destination and the gap in time between one episode ending and another starting. Each of these steps is based on assumptions which need testing. Successful linkage is also dependent on completeness of data in all the required fields. Data within the HES system are collected by year and not linked between years. Given the dependence of linkage on availability of data on the start and finish of the episode, some episodes starting in a previous year or ending in the following year may get excluded from indicators for a particular year.

As linkage is done from a national file containing all episodes, irrespective of place of treatment, such linkage deals with movements of patients across boundaries. For example, if a patient is discharged from one hospital in one district and is subsequently readmitted to another hospital in another district, this will be picked up by such linkage. Similarly, for a district-based indicator, all episodes for residents of a district will be part of the indicator, including those where treatment took place outside the district. Successful cross-boundary linkage, however, is dependent on completeness of postal code data which are used to define the district of residence of a patient.

The rates have not been adjusted for differences between hospitals in the mix of patients based on types of illnesses, concurrent illnesses, severity of disease, seriousness of operation or numbers of operations as methods for assigning case-mix classifications to continuous inpatient spells have yet to be developed. In addition, the NHS does not collect data on disease severity. Deaths occurring after discharge from hospital are excluded as there is no linkage between hospital records and death registration data. The data are presented with hospitals grouped on the basis of type of hospital, in order to compare 'like' with 'like' as far as is possible. There is substantial variation between like hospitals in such death rates. The indicator has many limitations, explained within detailed technical specifications

Assessment of clinical and health outcomes

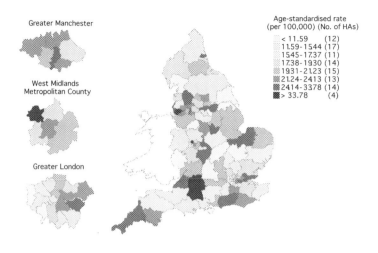

Figure 8.4 Hospital episode rates for diabetic ketoacidosis and coma. Directly standardised rates for females (all ages), year ending 31 March 1997. Crown copyright material from the NCHOD's Clinical and Health Outcomes Knowledge Base, reproduced with the permission of the Controller of Her Majesty's Stationery Office.

accompanying their publication.[7] They are still being refined and operation-specific indicators are under development. However, previous confidential inquiries into deaths after surgery have shown that some such deaths are associated with shortcomings in healthcare. The extent of observed variation cannot be ignored and needs further investigation.

Indicators reflecting outcome based on incidence of disease

There are few instances of data on population-based incidence of disease collected routinely. Examples include cancer registration and notifications of some infectious diseases. Figure 8.4[4] shows how data on hospitalisation have been used to assess population incidence of disease, and hence outcome. Diabetic ketoacidosis and coma are severe consequences of diabetes. When they occur they may reflect failure of control of diabetes. Patients with these conditions need hospitalisation. Postcode data may be used to relate each patient to a health authority of residence, and hence calculate the population incidence of these conditions. As with previous examples, there is a lot of variation between 'like' populations in conditions which are

123

potentially avoidable. The indicator is limited, firstly, because numbers are small and, secondly, as there may be problems with the quality of coding of clinical data, resulting in an incomplete indicator. Figure 8.5 shows variation between NHS Executive regional office populations in the incidence of high blood pressure. This indicator is based on analysis of data from the Health Survey for England.[8] Given the sample size, it is not possible to produce indicators at health authority level. The indicator is nevertheless useful. Not only does it show outcome of NHS care in terms of treated and controlled high blood pressure, it also acts as a proxy for future potential adverse outcome, in that some people with untreated or uncontrolled high blood pressure may go on to develop stroke.

Association between incidence and intervention

Some of the difficulties in attributing health end-points to specific healthcare interventions were explained earlier. It may still be useful to examine data on interventions and outcomes alongside each other as they may lead to more specific questions and issues for further investigation. Figure 8.6[9] shows survey-based data on oral health and

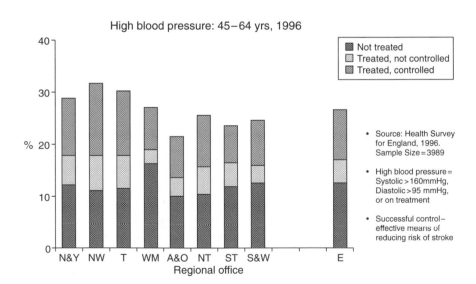

Figure 8.5 NHS success in reducing risk. This example shows the control of high blood pressure. Crown copyright material from the NCHOD's Clinical and Health Outcomes Knowledge Base, reproduced with the permission of the Controller of Her Majesty's Stationery Office.

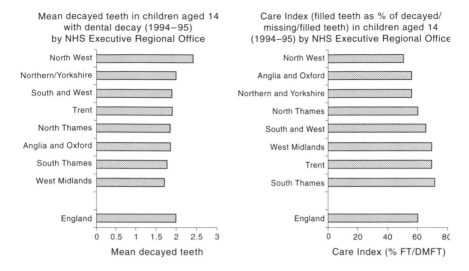

Figure 8.6 Success in reducing level of disease and its effective treatment – example: oral health. Crown copyright material from the NCHOD's Clinical and Health Outcomes Knowledge Base, reproduced with the permission of the Controller of Her Majesty's Stationery Office.

the level of treatment among resident populations of NHS Executive Regional Offices. Alongside regional variation in both indicators, there does appear to be an inverse relationship between incidence and treatment.

Process as a proxy for outcome

The NHS has a policy to screen women aged 20–64 years for cervical cancer at least once every 5 years. Data on take-up of the service are collected as part of service monitoring and are collated nationally. Figure 8.7[10] shows variation between 'like' populations in the coverage of eligible populations by this service and may act as a proxy for future outcome. The actual outcome, in terms of prolonged survival through early detection of this treatable cancer, may take decades to manifest itself.

A proxy for improvement in quality of life

There is research-based evidence to show that hip replacement surgery, if used appropriately, leads to improvements in the quality of life through pain relief and improvement in mobility. The NHS does not collect data routinely on quality of life outcomes among the patients treated within it. However, data on the numbers of

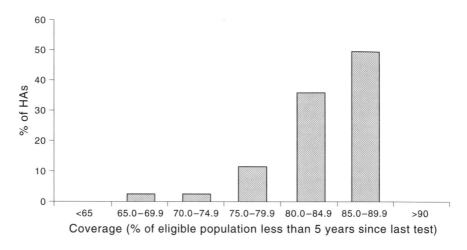

Figure 8.7 Cervical screening: coverage of target age group (25–64) by health authority, England, 31 March 1999. Crown copyright material from the Department of Health's bulletin on the Cervical Cancer Screening Programme, printed with the permission of the Controller of Her Majesty's Stationery Office.

operations carried out may be used as a proxy. Figure 8.8[4] shows variation in population rates of this operation as well as an association with the socio-economic characteristics of populations, based on the ONS area classification mentioned earlier. There is a suggestion that deprived populations appear to be getting relatively less of this potentially beneficial treatment. This would be even more apparent if data from the private healthcare sector were available as they would probably increase rates within populations classified at the more prosperous end of the spectrum. It is interesting to note the variation within groups of 'like' populations. In addition, there are no data on variation in incidence of hip joint problems, hence need for the surgery. There are no data on criteria for selection of patients for surgery, thresholds for treatment, appropriateness of the operation for individual patients, local waiting list initiatives, etc. and these may vary between populations.

Supplementing official statistics

The indicators described above suffer from the limitations of routine data as discussed. This is not surprising as the latter were not necessarily specified and collected for the purposes of monitoring outcomes. The indicators do, however, highlight areas meriting further local investigation, which may require additional local data

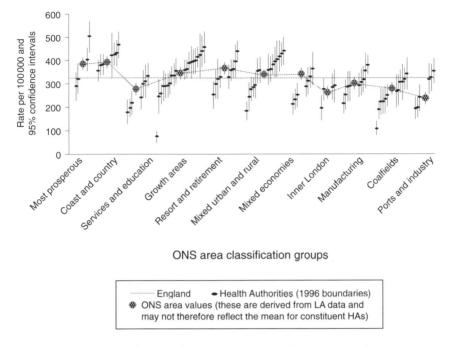

ONS area classification groups

----------- England   ● Health Authorities (1996 boundaries)
⊛ ONS area values (these are derived from LA data and
   may not therefore reflect the mean for constituent HAs)

Figure 8.8 Primary total hip replacement rates. Directly standardised rates for females (aged 65+), year ending 31 March 1997. Crown copyright material from the NCHOD's Clinical and Health Outcomes Knowledge Base, reproduced with the permission of the Controller of Her Majesty's Stationery Office.

collection. Over the years, the CHOU and the NCHOD have commissioned and undertaken development work to show how supplementary data could be collected and used locally. The results of the development work can be found within the *Clinical and Health Outcomes Knowledge Base.*

Specification and piloting of new indicators

One example is the work of ten working groups set up to advise on new health outcome indicators, some of which may require new data collection at local level to supplement indicators based on routine data. The topics covered by the working groups include asthma, breast cancer, cataract, diabetes mellitus, fractured proximal femur, myocardial infarction, normal pregnancy and childbirth, severe mental illness, stroke and urinary incontinence. Each working group was tasked to make recommendations on 'ideal indicators' defined as statistical measures of what should be known and realistically could be known about the outcomes of the condition

127

in routine clinical practice. The groups had members who brought together the perspectives of all the relevant clinical professions plus patients, NHS managers, policy makers, researchers and others as appropriate and were supported by a number of technical institutions. The reports of all the working groups have now been published. The stroke report,[11] for example, contains detailed specifications for 24 indicators and their variants covering aspects such as reduction/avoidance of first and subsequent stroke, reduction of death from stroke, reduction/avoidance of complications from stroke and improving function and well-being after stroke. Many of the indicators in the reports have been piloted to test their feasibility, either using enhanced routine datasets such as the Oxford Record Linkage Study or new local data collection. The Oxford Record Linkage Study links person-based data on hospitalisation, mortality and various other aspects as appropriate.[12]

Mapping of indicators on to the NHS Performance Assessment Framework

Existing indicators in the *Knowledge Base* have been brought together and mapped on to the *NHS Performance Assessment Framework*[3] for 33 health topics or clinical conditions at present. New indicators will be mapped as they are included in the *Knowledge Base*. Box 8.1 shows for one condition, stroke, how existing and potential indicators might give a more rounded view of service performance.

Local follow-up work

Following a survey on how health authorities (HA) in England were using population health outcome indicators, a series of case studies on work undertaken at HA level to follow up indicator values of concern were commissioned. Twenty-six case studies have now been published[13] and cover aspects such as why a particular clinical area was selected for study; further information that was required; data validity studies; results of the studies; changes which were made; how changes are going to be monitored; resource implications; practical lessons learnt; and conclusions. The full reports are available within the *Knowledge Base*. Table 8.2 is an illustrative summary of some of the case studies and their findings showing, for example, how high death rates from stroke in one health authority, Wandsworth, led to such a study and subsequent changes in service policy.

Box 8.1 Mapping the compendium of clinical health indicators to the NHS Performance Assessment Framework – stroke

⇒ **Health improvement**
  - Cigarette smoking prevalence
  - Food energy derived from saturated fatty acids
  - Food energy derived from total fat
  - Alcohol consumption above sensible levels
  - Body Mass Index > 30 kg/^{2}m
  - Mean population levels of blood pressure
  - Population death rates and years of life lost

⇒ **Fair access**
  - Systematic variation in intervention rates
  - Systematic variation in outcomes

⇒ **Effective delivery of appropriate healthcare**
  ◆ *Known to be effective (evidence-based)*
    - [Aspirin therapy 6 months after stroke]
    - [Anti-coagulant therapy for atrial fibrillation]
  ◆ *Appropriate to need*
    - [Multiprofessional input to care after stroke]
  ◆ *Timely*
    - [Swallowing assessment within 24 hours of stroke]
  ◆ *Compliance with standards*
    - Blood pressure recorded by GP in previous 5 yrs
    - [Body Mass Index recorded by GP previously]
    - [Alcohol consumption recorded by GP previously]
    - Discharged to usual residence within 56 days
  ◆ *Service organisation*
    - [Implementation of Service Framework]

⇒ **Efficiency**
  ◆ *Cost per unit of care*
    - Average length of emergency hospital episode

⇒ **Patient/Carer experience**
    - [Patients'/carers' knowledge of available services]
    - [Patient satisfaction with treatment and outcome]
    - [Carer burden 7 months after stroke]

⇒ **Health outcome of NHS care**
  ◆ *NHS success in reducing level of risk*
    - Prevalence of untreated/uncontrolled high blood pressure
    - [Median/inter-quartile range of BP recorded by GP]
    - [Hypertensive patients with GP record of high blood pressure]
  ◆ *NHS success in reducing level of disease and impairment*
    - [Population-based incidence of stroke]
    - Emergency hospitalisation for stroke
  ◆ *NHS success in reducing adverse consequences of treatment*
    - [Incidence of pressure sores following stroke]
    - Emergency readmission within 30 days of discharge
  ◆ *NHS success in restoring function and improving quality of life of patients/carers*
    - [Aphasia 6 months after stroke]

- Discharge to usual residence within 56 days
- [% living in usual residence 6 months after stroke]
- [Barthel index at discharge and 6 months after stroke]
- [Outdoor mobility 6 months after stroke]
- [Social functioning 6 months after stroke]
- [Depression 6 months after stroke]
◆ *NHS success in reducing premature deaths*
- Death rates among various age groups
- Case fatality rates in hospital
- [Case fatality rates in community]

Note: Indicators in [ ] are potential indicators. National comparative data are available for the rest.

New developments: Information for Health Strategy

The limitations of existing routine data have been acknowledged by the government for many years and strategies have been developed to overcome some of these, as far as is feasible. The most recent strategy document *Information for Health*[14] was published in 1998 and covers plans for developments in information management and technology within the NHS for the period up to 2005. The strategy includes, for example, aspects such as the development of structured person-based electronic patient records, an NHS–wide electronic network and a common language for health. These would make possible the production of comparative data on many of the 'ideal' indicators recommended in the ten working group reports and others as well as enhanced and more appropriate monitoring of health outcomes at local level using routine data.

Conclusion

The indicators described in this chapter are not precise measures of outcome but are indicative of what may or may not have been achieved in the context of stated objectives. They also raise questions and issues for further investigation. For example, the observed variation in indicator values, both between as well as within groups of similar populations, suggests that achievements are not optimal. The best values achieved show what is possible in reality as it is actually being achieved. Such values may help to set more realistic targets than those based on extrapolation from the research

Table 8.2 Improving health outcomes: case studies

Area	Condition	Findings	Action
South Lancashire	Breast cancer	High incidence	Raise awareness Screening Quality of treatment
Wandsworth	Stroke	Inequity of access Variation in rehabilitation Variation in community care Need for education	New framework for services
Barking and Havering	Diabetes	Variety of problems	Register Shared care guidelines Foot clinic Children's nurse Day centre
Sheffield	Coronary heart disease	Angina survey (16 000) Mismatch between need and access	New policies for service access
East Anglia Region	Hip fracture	Variation in: deaths pressure sores DVT prophylaxis antibiotic prophylaxis time to surgery early mobilisation	Service changes

Source: McColl *et al.*, University of Southampton. Crown copyright material from the NCHOD's Clinical and Health Outcomes Knowledge Base, reproduced with the permission of the Controller of Her Majesty's Stationery Office.

literature, where the populations being studied may have been subject to selection. Performance, over time, could be judged on the basis of both reduction in variation between populations as well as movement towards the best values achieved. Despite their limitations, official statistics may go some way towards helping the NHS and others judge the extent to which the NHS has been successful in its attempts to use its resources to achieve the greatest possible improvement in health. Such judgement may be enhanced by additional supplementary data collection.

Note

The work of the National Centre for Health Outcomes Development is funded by the Department of Health. All views expressed are those of the author and not necessarily of the Department of Health.

References

1 NHS Executive Communications Unit (1996) *A Guide to the National Health Service*. Health Publications Unit, Heywood, Lancs.
2 Department of Health (1998) *A First Class Service: quality in the new NHS*. Department of Health, London.
3 NHS Executive (1999) *The NHS Performance Assessment Framework*. NHS Executive, Leeds.
4 National Centre for Health Outcomes Development (1999) *Clinical and Health Outcomes Knowledge Base*. National Centre for Health Outcomes Development, London/Oxford.
5 Lakhani A (1994) *Central Health Outcomes Unit*. Department of Health, London.
6 NHS Executive (1999) *Quality and Performance in the New NHS: high level performance indicators and clinical indicators*. NHS Executive, Leeds.
7 Public Health Development Unit (1999) *Quality and Performance in the NHS: clinical indicators technical supplement*. NHS Executive, Leeds.
8 Prescott-Clarke P, Primatesta P (eds) (1998) *Health Survey for England 1996. Vol. 1: Findings*. The Stationery Office, London.
9 Department of Health (1997) *Public Health Common Data Set 1996*. National Institute of Epidemiology, Surrey.
10 Department of Health (1999) *Cervical Cancer Screening Programme, England: 1998–99*. Bulletin 1999/32. Department of Health, London.
11 Rudd A, Goldacre M, Amess M *et al.* (1999) *Health Outcome Indicators: stroke. Report of a working group to the Department of Health*. National Centre for Health Outcomes Development, Oxford.
12 Gill L, Goldacre M, Simmons H *et al.* (1993) Computerised linking of medical records: methodological guidelines. *Journal of Epidemiology and Community Health.* **47**: 316–19.
13 McColl A, Roderick P, Gabbay J (1997) *Improving Health Outcomes. Case studies on how English health authorities use population based health outcome assessments*. The Wessex Institute for Health Research and Development, Southampton.
14 NHS Executive (1998) *Information for Health: an information strategy for the modern NHS 1998–2005: a national strategy for local implementation*. Health Service Circular HSC 98/168, Leeds.

9 Birth and maternity statistics

Alison Macfarlane

Introduction

This chapter describes the systems from which birth and maternity data can be derived for use at a local level. These are the civil registration of births, the notification of births and hospital-based data collection systems. The way these systems operate and the extent to which they can be used differ between the four countries of the UK. The chapter closes with an overview of the proposals for change which are under development at the time of writing.

Of course, these are not the only routinely collected data which are relevant to birth and maternity care. Data are collected about facilities and staffing of the maternity services and about the socio-economic context in which childbirth occurs. A much wider range of data is reviewed in the first volume of *Birth Counts: statistics of pregnancy and childbirth*.[1] The second volume of *Birth Counts* is a compilation of data aggregated at a national level with some regional data.[2]

Birth registration

Birth registration is the oldest source of data about births. Like death registration, described in Chapter 2, registration of live births started in 1838 in England and Wales, 1855 in Scotland and 1864 in Ireland. The primary reason for setting up systems for registering births, marriages and deaths was to provide civil documents to record the events for legal purposes.[3,4] Nevertheless, the General Register Office (GRO), set up to oversee registration in England and Wales, developed a high profile statistical department under the leadership of William Farr, who was a prominent figure in the nineteenth century statistical movement.[5] When the GROs for Scotland and Ireland were set up, they too started to compile and publish statistics. For a variety of reasons, the initial legislation did not cover stillbirths.[1] Stillbirth registration was introduced in 1927 in England and Wales, 1939 in Scotland and 1961 in Northern Ireland.

Initially, fetal deaths at 28 or more completed weeks of gestation had to be registered as stillbirths, but the limit was lowered to 24 weeks on 1 October 1992.

From the very outset, producing statistics for local areas was an important part of the work of the general register offices. The groups of parishes, known as 'poor law unions', established for the administration of the 1834 Poor Law were used as a basis for organising birth and death registration and data were compiled for these areas. In 1911, new technology, in the form of equipment for sorting and counting punched cards, made it possible to tabulate data for the local government districts which had been established in the latter half of the nineteenth century.[6] From then onwards, birth and death data have been compiled and published annually for local government districts. Since 1974, when separate districts were established for administration of the NHS, data have been routinely tabulated and published for these areas as well.

Not surprisingly the organisations responsible for analysing the data from birth registration have changed over the years. After the partition of Ireland, a separate GRO for Northern Ireland was established in 1922. In 1970 the GRO for England and Wales became part of the Office of Population Censuses and Surveys (OPCS) until 1996 when OPCS merged with the Central Statistical Office to form the Office for National Statistics (ONS). This is now responsible for birth registration for England and Wales and the data derived from it, along with the wide range of other data described in Chapter 2. The Northern Ireland Statistics and Research Agency (NISRA) was also formed in 1996 and its work includes demographic analysis of data collected by the GRO for Northern Ireland.

Data collected at birth registration

Under the legislation in force in the countries of the UK, a live birth must be registered with the local registrar within 42 days of occurrence. Stillbirths must be registered within three months in England, Wales and Northern Ireland and 21 days in Scotland. Usually births are registered by the baby's parents, but they can also be registered by another next of kin or by the midwife or doctor present at the birth. To register a stillbirth, the informant normally produces a medical certificate, completed by a doctor or midwife who was present at the birth or who examined the body. If the parents are not married, they can register the birth jointly or the mother can register it on her own. These are described as 'joint registration' and 'sole registration' in published statistics for England and Wales. No distinction is made between categories of birth outside marriage in Scotland and Northern Ireland.

At registration, the registrar asks the informant the mother's name, her usual address, her date and country of birth and the place where the birth occurred. For births within marriage and jointly registered births outside marriage in England and Wales, the father's occupation and date of birth are recorded. At sole registrations, the mother's occupation is recorded. Since 1986, all other mothers have had the option of recording their own occupation as well as the father's. In Scotland, the mother's occupation is recorded for all births outside marriage and the father's for births within marriage.

Under the Population (Statistics) Acts of 1938 and 1960, the number of previous live and stillbirths to the current or any previous husband is recorded, for births within marriage only. This differs markedly from the definition of parity used in clinical practice, which is simply the number of previous live and stillbirths for the mother. The question asked at birth registration and the legislation underpinning it date back to the 1930s when attitudes were different and over 95% of births were within marriage, so the difference was minimal. OPCS made proposals for change in 1990, but was unable to implement them at the time, in the absence of primary legislation.[7]

Traditionally, the local registrar recorded the information collected at birth registration on a 'draft entry' form and forwarded it to the relevant GRO. By the late 1990s, most local register offices in England and Wales were using computers with standard software and now forward the data on diskettes.

At the time of writing, local registrars in England and Wales allocate the baby's NHS number and send this, together with a copy of the draft entry, to the local director of public health. In practice, since 1991, the draft entry has been sent to the local community trust. In England and Wales, the community trust extracts the baby's birthweight from the birth notification, which is described later. It passes the information to the local registrar, who adds it to the baby's draft entry before forwarding it to the ONS. For stillbirths, birthweight and gestational age are stated on the certificate. The ONS does not currently have access to data about the gestational age at live

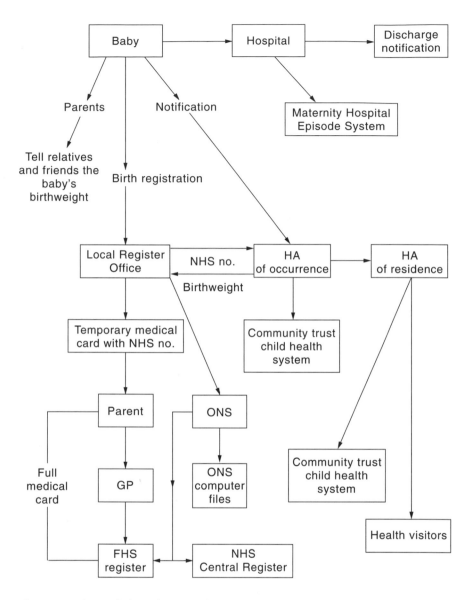

Figure 9.1 Flows of data about live births in England, 1999.

birth. The data flows for live births are illustrated in Figure 9.1. It has been recognised for some time that this procedure is somewhat cumbersome. A number of reviews, the latest of which are under way at the time of writing and outlined at the end of the chapter, may lead to changes which are long overdue.

Accessing birth registration data

Data from birth registration are published annually in *Birth Statistics, England and Wales, Series FM1,* and *Annual Reports* of the Registrar General for Scotland and the Registrar General, Northern Ireland. All contain tabulations of live births at national level. Live births are tabulated by council and health board area in the report for Scotland. The Northern Ireland report contains some tables of live births for all administrative areas while others are at health and social services board level.

Birth Statistics, Series FM1 contains detailed tabulations of births in England and Wales by parents' ages and marital status, the father's social class and the mother's country of birth along with analyses of fertility. Most of these are for England and Wales as a whole, with only a few tables for NHS and other regions. Since April 1997, England has been split into nine government office regions. Data for local authority and health authority areas are published in less detail in *Key Population and Vital Statistics, Series VS.* In addition, the Department of Health includes some birth registration data for England in *Health and Personal Social Services Statistics for England.* Similar data for Wales appear in *Health Statistics Wales,* published by the National Assembly for Wales, which succeeded the Welsh Office in July 1999.

Although the ONS is taking steps to speed up production, these annual volumes tend to emerge a year or more after the end of the year to which the data relate. Other data are circulated more quickly. Up to 1998, provisional data were published earlier in the *Monitor* series, but now appear in ONS quarterly journals *Population Trends* and *Health Statistics Quarterly.*

More detailed unpublished tables are produced for local areas. These date back to the nineteenth century when they were sent to Medical Officers of Health. Before 1981 they were known as 'SD' tabulations, reflecting their origins as tables circulated to 'sanitary districts', the old name for local authorities.

In 1981, OPCS reorganised these tabulations into the *Vital Statistics* (VS) series. Three contain birth data. The VS1 vital statistics summary contains populations, numbers of births and deaths and fertility rates, for local and health authority areas. They also make comparisons with the relevant regions and with England and Wales as a whole. The VS2 birth statistics summaries are for the same areas and show numbers of births by age of mother, marital status, number of previous live births to current or previous husbands, birthweight and type of institution in which the birth occurred. Data at ward level in the VS4 tabulations include numbers of live births and stillbirths. The ONS sends each local health authority the VS tabulations for its area as paper printouts, usually within six months of the year to which they relate. In addition, the whole set can be purchased as *DVS tabulations* on CD-ROM.

Special arrangements have been made to enable health authorities to buy computer files of individual records of registrations of births and deaths of their residents and those of surrounding areas. These extracts were originally supplied on paper by registrars to local directors of public health under the National Health Service Act 1977 and earlier legislation dating back to the nineteenth century. The ONS provides these in two forms.

The public health mortality file and the public health birth file contain the details recorded at registration which are on the public record, including names and addresses. These files also include codes for some items, such as the cause of death. They include not only births and deaths of health authority residents, but also births and deaths occurring within the district to people resident elsewhere. The ONS can provide these weekly or monthly on disk, giving health authorities access to data which are up to the minute, although not fully quality assured. The data can be used for event linkage, audit, screening, confidential enquiry into stillbirths and infant deaths, monitoring trends in the local population, list cleaning in the NHS or social services and producing small area statistics.

Health authorities which do not want to analyse birth and death data more often than once a year, for example for annual public health reports, can buy annual birth and death extracts. In 2000, these extracts cost £60 for each health authority. The annual cost of the weekly public health *mortality* file was £3300 and that of the monthly file was £3000. The public health *births* file was £1000 per annum for the weekly version and £850 per annum for the monthly version.

Under the Act mentioned above, these extracts are available only to health authorities. Other users can request an ad hoc purchase of files containing suitably anonymised birth and death individual records.

Stillbirths and infant mortality

Although ONS' *Birth Statistics, Series FM1* contains some data about stillbirths in England and Wales, more detailed analyses are published in *Mortality Statistics, Childhood, Infant and Perinatal, Series DH3*. This now contains only one regional analysis. A basic table of stillbirth and infant mortality rates for district and NHS regions was published annually in the *Monitor* series up to 1998. From 1999 onwards it has appeared in ONS' journal *Health Statistics Quarterly*. Similar data are subsequently published in *Key Population and Vital Statistics, Series VS*. More detailed data for local authority and health authority areas can be found in the VS5 infant and perinatal mortality tables. These are available as DVS5 tables on CD-ROM.

In 1975, OPCS started to link data collected about the deaths of babies aged under one year with data collected at birth registration. As a result, tabulations of infant mortality rates by mother's age and country of birth, father's social class and the type of institution in which the baby was born have been published annually. In 1993, at the time of the computer redevelopment referred to in Chapter 2, this was extended. Data about the death of any child born from 1993 onward are linked to birth registration data. Initially, tabulations at the level of NHS regions and health authorities were published routinely, but this is no longer the case. As with unlinked births and deaths, it is possible to obtain extracts of anonymised individual records for further analysis.

In Scotland, tabulations of stillbirth and infant mortality rates for local areas can be found in *Scottish Health Statistics* published annually by the Information and Statistic Divisions (ISD). Linkage is made between registration data and the SMR2 maternity discharge data, which are described later. This is used to produce the tables published by ISD in the *Scottish Stillbirth and Infant Death Report*, which includes some tables for health board areas.

Local stillbirth and infant mortality rates for Northern Ireland are published in the *Annual Report* of the Registrar General. No linkage is made between birth and infant death registration.

Coding and classifying the certified causes of stillbirth and infant death

As with deaths of any age, the certified causes of stillbirth and infant death are coded as described in Chapter 2, using the International

Classification of Diseases. As mentioned there, new forms of certificate for certifying causes of stillbirths and neonatal deaths were introduced in England and Wales but not Scotland or Northern Ireland in 1986. There are currently no plans to introduce these forms of certificate in Scotland or in Northern Ireland.

The certificates used in England and Wales are shown in Figures 9.2 and 9.3. Their introduction posed problems in deciding how to group and classify the conditions mentioned on the different parts of the certificate, as it is no longer possible to derive a single underlying cause of death. Classifications derived from Jonathan Wigglesworth's pathophysiological classification have been used for coding the conditions on the stillbirth and neonatal death certificates.[8–10] In the published tables, the groups are described as 'ONS cause groups'.

Confidential enquiries

Since 1992, in England, Wales and Northern Ireland, the Confidential Enquiry into Stillbirths and Deaths in Infancy (CESDI) has collected data about fetal deaths from 20 completed weeks of gestation and deaths in the first year after live birth. Each year defined subsets of deaths have been subjected to confidential review by regional panels, based in the 14 former NHS regions of England and in Wales and Northern Ireland. An annual report is published about the Enquiry as a whole.[11] National reports are published for Wales and Northern Ireland and most English regions usually publish their own report.

CESDI is based largely on the model of the Confidential Enquiry into Maternal Deaths. This took its present form in 1952 in England and Wales, 1965 in Scotland and 1964 in Northern Ireland. From the 3-year period 1985–87 onwards, data from all four countries have been published in a common report.[12]

Notification of births

Birth notification was instituted as part of a wider policy of establishing maternal and child welfare schemes during the first decade of the twentieth century. These involved visiting new mothers soon after birth to offer help and advice. With parents having up to six weeks to register a birth, and most births occurring at home, it could take some time for the copy of the registration to reach the Medical Officer of Health and then the staff of the scheme. Therefore the Notification of

MEDICAL CERTIFICATE OF STILL-BIRTH

(Births and Deaths Registration Act 1953, S 11(1), as amended by the Population (Statistics) Act 1960)
(Form prescribed by the Registration of Births and Deaths Regulations 1987)

SB 806321

To be given only in respect of a child which has issued forth from its mother after the 24th week of pregnancy and which did not at any time after being completely expelled from its mother breathe or show any other signs of life.

Registered at
Entry No.

*I was present at the still-birth of a $\dfrac{\text{*male}}{\text{*female}}$ child born

*I have examined the body of a $\dfrac{\text{*male}}{\text{*female}}$ child which I am informed and believe was born

on .... day of .... 19 .... to ....
(NAME OF MOTHER)

at ....
(PLACE OF BIRTH)

†{ 1 The certified cause of death has been confirmed by post-mortem.
     2 Post-mortem information may be available later.
     3 Post-mortem not being held.

Weight of fetus .... grams
Estimated duration of pregnancy
State (a) the number of weeks of delivery ....
       (b) When the child died
                                    (i) before labour*
                                    (ii) during labour*
                                    (iii) not known*

**Strike out the words which do not apply.*
†*Ring appropriate digit.*

CAUSE OF DEATH

SPECIMEN

a. Main diseases or conditions in fetus

b. Other diseases or conditions in fetus ....

c. Main maternal diseases or conditions affecting fetus ....

d. Other maternal diseases or conditions affecting fetus ....

e. Other relevant causes ....

I hereby certify that (i) the child was not born alive, and
                      (ii) to the best of my knowledge and belief the cause of death and the estimated duration of
                           pregnancy of the mother were as stated above.

Signature ....   Date ....

Qualification as registered by General Medical Council, or }
  Registered No. as Registered Midwife.   } ....

Address ....

For still-births in hospital: please give the name of the consultant responsible for the care of the mother ....

THIS IS NOT AN AUTHORITY FOR BURIAL OR CREMATION [SEE OVER]

Figure 9.2 Certificate used in 2000 for certifying stillbirths. (© Crown copyright. Reproduced with the permission of the controller of HMSO. *Source*: ONS.)

Births Extension Act of 1915 required that all births were notified to the local Medical Officer of Health within 36 hours.

Despite all that has changed in the intervening years, this requirement still exists. Although it was initially envisaged that parents would notify births, this is now usually, but not necessarily, done by the midwife attending the birth. In theory, the notification goes to the Director of Public Health, but since the introduction of the 'purchaser provider split' in 1991, it is usually sent to the local community trust.

The purpose of notification is to alert health visitors of the birth so that they can do postnatal visits and developmental checks. Community trusts run the child health surveillance systems used to

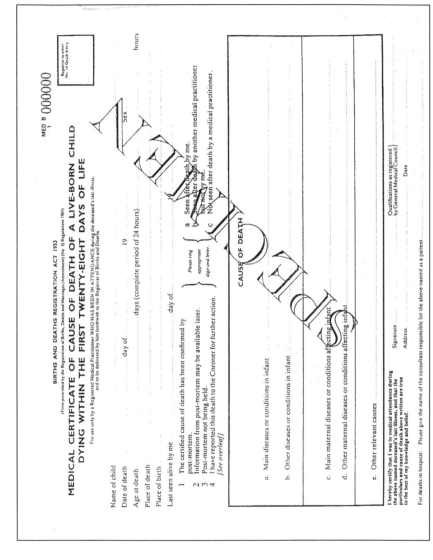

Figure 9.3 Certificate used in 2000 for certifying deaths within the first 28 days of life. (© Crown copyright. Reproduced with the permission of the controller of HMSO. *Source*: ONS.)

administer appointments for immunisation and developmental checks and monitor the extent to which they take place. Notification forms are used to set up children's records on surveillance systems. The data collected vary from district to district. As was mentioned earlier, they include birthweight. In England and Wales, this is passed to the registrar of births and deaths once the draft entry is received with the baby's NHS number.

Notification of congenital anomalies

Most districts in England and Wales also use birth notifications as a source of information about congenital anomalies apparent at birth, which they notify to the ONS. The system for monitoring anomalies in England and Wales was set up in 1964 following the birth of children with major limb malformations to women who had taken the drug thalidomide in pregnancy. Each month the ONS compares the numbers of particular types of anomalies reported from each district with recent trends reported from that district and informs the health authority of any increases.[13]

Under-reporting has always been a problem with this system, despite a number of attempts to improve it. The system originally applied to anomalies detected within ten days of birth, although not all of these were notified. By definition anomalies which do not become apparent until later, for example cardiovascular anomalies, could not be recorded. Since 1 January 1995, the upper time limit no longer applies. A review in 1995 made a number of other recommendations for improvements.[14] Perhaps the most important of these was that if there was a local register of anomalies, data from this should be forwarded to the ONS, rather than duplicating effort by using parallel sets of notifications. This is now beginning to happen and the ONS is working with local registers through the British Isles Network of Congenital Anomaly Registers (BINOCAR). The ONS publishes the data annually in *Congenital Anomaly Statistics, Series MB3*.

Scotland and Northern Ireland have separate notification systems. In Scotland, data about congenital anomalies come from three sources, the SMR2 maternity record, SMR1 and SMR11 records of hospital inpatient stays by babies and the stillbirth and neonatal death records. ISD publishes the data in *Congenital Malformations in Scotland*. In Northern Ireland, congenital anomalies are monitored by the Regional Medical Genetics Centre at Belfast City Hospital and published in the *Annual Report of Chief Medical Officer for Northern Ireland*.

Child health systems

Most child health surveillance systems were designed from the late 1960s onward as operational systems. Initially they were designed for scheduling immunisations and they were then developed for pre-school and school health surveillance. They were largely consolidated into a national system from the mid 1970s onwards.[15] Alternative systems were produced from the late 1980s onwards. It is not easy to use child health systems to link data about individual children and derive statistics. Apart from special projects, such as the Regionally Integrated Child Health System (RICHS) project in the former North East Thames Region, they have not been widely used in England or Scotland for data analysis or the production of tables, and their potential remains unexploited. It is difficult to define cohorts of children in a mobile population and there are problems about ensuring completeness and quality of data.[16,17] Developments have taken place in Wales and Northern Ireland, however.

In Wales, the Welsh Health Common Services Agency, now known as Health Solutions, Wales has defined a common dataset to supplement data already collected at birth notification.[18] It has established a national database of data derived from birth notification and uses it for local and national analyses. The next step is to redevelop child health systems and move towards a national database linking subsequent developmental tests and diagnoses to information collected at birth.

In Northern Ireland, each of the four health and social services boards maintains a child health system and produces analyses of data from birth notifications. Data are aggregated for the province as a whole. It is unclear how these systems will develop in the future, as proposals have been made to abolish the four boards and replace them with a single board for Northern Ireland. It is unclear at the time of writing how these proposals will affect data collection.

Child health surveillance systems have the potential to collect data about morbidity in childhood and link them to circumstances at birth. This potential has yet to be realised. Comparisons with registers of children with cerebral palsy show that it is under-reported in child health systems.[19,20] This means that improvements are needed in the completeness and quality of the data. As child health systems are not primarily designed for data analysis, gaps and inconsistencies may not be readily identified.

Hospital-based data derived from case notes and clinical systems

There is a long tradition of individual midwives and hospitals collecting data about their practice, but data collection has not developed in a consistent way. In her *Introductory Notes on Lying-in Institutions*, published in 1871, Florence Nightingale tried to compare data about maternal mortality rates among women delivering in various institutions or at home with care from their 'outdoor departments'.[21] She complained that the institutions did not keep their statistics according to a 'uniform plan' and recommended a common set of data items to be used for maternity records. At the beginning of the twenty-first century, the lack of consensus she observed has not yet been resolved and still is a major problem. It makes comparisons between data for different areas and between local and national rates difficult, except perhaps in Scotland. The problems with current maternity systems arise out of the way they developed in the latter half of the twentieth century.

The first attempts to collect hospital data at a national level were made during the Second World War. These set a precedent for the Hospital In-Patient Enquiry (HIPE) set up in 1949 in England and Wales and similar systems in Scotland and Northern Ireland. From 1952 onwards, HIPE was based on data from a 10% sample of discharges from hospitals in England and Wales. If the discharge was from a maternity department, additional data items were collected about the care given. These were analysed separately as Maternity HIPE.

In the 1960s, Wales and NHS regions in England started to use systems of Hospital Activity Analysis (HAA) containing data about all discharges, except of mental health patients. HAA data were analysed locally and 10% of samples were extracted for national analysis in HIPE. A system of Maternity HAA was developed, but was not generally accepted and it covered only about a third of births in England and Wales.[22,23] A number of computerised local and regional maternity information systems grew up and samples were extracted from these for Maternity HIPE. Between them these systems covered about one-third of births. Data about the remaining third of discharges were collected by extracting data from case notes to fill in paper forms.

Following the review by the Steering Group on Health Services Information in the early 1980s, HAA evolved into the Hospital Episode Statistics (HES), described in Chapter 4.[24-26] If one or more babies are born during an episode of admitted patient care, there should be an HES record for each baby, with a 'maternity tail' appended containing the 19 items of the maternity dataset.[25,26]

Although Maternity HES got underway some 18 months after the main HES system, many records of deliveries lacked 'maternity tails' while others had 'maternity tails' containing no data. Overall, there were maternity tails with data for around two thirds of deliveries in England.[26]

For some years, data were not published because of their poor quality. Eventually, the Department of Health (DoH) published a statistical bulletin containing time trends in variables such as induction rates and method of delivery, along with regional and other analyses for the financial year 1994/95.[19] It has several tables showing data such as induction and operative delivery by trust and these reveal clearly those who submitted no data. They include some trusts which are known to collect and publish good quality data elsewhere in their own reports and in journal articles.[27] The DoH plans to issue further bulletins of data from Maternity HES in an annual series.

Not surprisingly, the bulletin contains a full discussion of data quality and coverage. After the coverage of Maternity HES rose from 57% of births in England in 1989/90 to 78% in 1992/93, it actually fell back to 67% in 1994/95.[26] Unlike the rest of HES, Maternity HES is intended to include births outside hospital and those in non-NHS hospitals. In 1994/95, it included records of only 28% of the registered births at home in England and fewer than 200 of the estimated 3500 deliveries in private hospitals.

A number of factors are likely to have contributed to this unsatisfactory situation, some of them being inherited from Maternity HIPE. A survey of NHS maternity units in 1997 showed that many had maternity computer systems which were not linked to their hospital's patient administration system, while others did not hold maternity data in a computer system.[28] As HES relies on sending data from patient administration systems through the NHS-wide clearing service, it will not capture maternity data unless there is better linkage between existing systems and facilities are provided to enter maternity data items into computer systems in the first place.

Although HES is very unreliable as a source of local maternity data, the bulletin can, when used with care, show national trends, such as rising caesarean section rates and the shift from forceps to ventouse for assisted delivery.[26] This means that if reliable data are available locally, they can be compared with national data from Maternity HES.

The recommendations of the Steering Group on Health Services Information were also implemented in Wales and Northern Ireland. Each of these countries has a system similar to HES. In Wales the system is called Patient Episode Data for Wales (PEDW). Checks made by the Welsh Health Common Services Agency showed that in 1997 just under 79% of deliveries generated a PEDW record and only one-third of these contained a maternity tail.[18] This was cited as a reason for developing the alternative data collection system based on birth notification. In Northern Ireland, very few of the delivery records in the Hospital In-Patients System have maternity tails with data, so they are not published.

Because of this situation, there are no national statistics about maternity care in Wales or Northern Ireland. The only country of the UK with reliable maternity statistics is Scotland. Since 1969, the SMR2 maternity discharge sheet has been used to collect data about hospital births in Scotland. By 1975, 96% of hospitals were covered and coverage has been virtually complete since then. From the early 1990s, the system was extended to the small numbers of home births, although not all were included by the end of the decade. Data both for Scotland as a whole and for individual health boards are published annually in *Scottish Health Statistics*. As mentioned earlier, the data are also linked with registration and other data and used in the *Scottish Stillbirths and Infant Death Report* and in special analyses. Data for the first 20 years were published in a special ISD report *Births in Scotland 1975–1995*.[29]

Data about all children born, not just those admitted to special or intensive care, are collected on SMR11 records. Coverage was virtually complete by 1981. As was mentioned earlier, SMR11 records are also used, together with data from the SMR1 system which covers all hospital stays apart from maternity, to collate data about congenital anomalies among children born in Scotland.

The system as a whole was revised for use with the 10th revision of the International Classification of Diseases (ICD10) and is now known as Core Patient Profile Information in Scottish Hospitals (COPPISH).

Future developments

Even when complemented with the other data described in *Birth Counts,* the picture at the end of the twentieth century is uneven and there are many gaps in the data.[1] All four countries of the UK have good quality data from birth registration, but only Wales and Northern Ireland make concerted attempts to use data from birth notification. Scotland is the only country with reliable data about maternity care.

Nevertheless, this book goes to press at a time when at least some of the problems have been recognised and a few attempts to tackle them are underway. Information strategies for England, Wales and Scotland were published in 1998 and 1999, although it is not immediately clear what impact they will have or how successful they will be in solving the problems identified here.[30-32] Nevertheless, a number of initiatives are already underway.

The first, arising out of *Information for Health*, the strategy for England, is the Maternity Care Data Project, which aims to have standardised and consistent recording of data by April 2003.[33] It overlaps with two other initiatives in England and Wales. The first is the issuing of NHS numbers at birth.[34] Pressure for this arose particularly from neonatologists who care for babies whose NHS numbers have yet to be allocated but wish to use them as an aid to monitoring subsequent morbidity in babies who are very ill at birth.

The second is the much wider review of civil registration. A consultation took place at the end of 1999. Proposals for greater use of information technology received strong support, and work began in 2000 on a policy document.

Meanwhile further developments are taking place in the use of child health system data in Wales and work is also being done in Scotland. Now that the Northern Ireland Assembly is established, proposals for reorganisation are being considered, and these may have an impact on statistical systems.

Thus although many problems remain, there is ground for limited optimism. Meanwhile, for people who need to use birth and maternity statistics, it is important to make the best use of the many data available, as well as trying to bring about the improvements which are needed.

Acknowledgements

Thanks to Lesz Lancucki of the Department of Health and Tim Devis, Doug Newbiggin, Nirupa Dattani and Vera Ruddock of the Office for National Statistics for commenting on earlier drafts. The author is funded by the Department of Health.

References

1   Macfarlane AJ and Mugford M (2000) *Birth Counts: statistics of pregnancy and childbirth. Vol. 1. Text.* The Stationery Office, London.
2   Macfarlane AJ, Mugford M, Henderson J *et al.* (2000) *Birth Counts: statistics of pregnancy and childbirth. Vol. 2. Tables.* The Stationery Office, London.
3   Higgs E (1996) A cuckoo in the nest? The origins of civil registration and state medical statistics in England and Wales. *Continuity and Change.* **11**(1): 115–34.
4   Nissel M. (1987) *People Count: a history of the General Register Office.* HMSO, London.
5   Eyler JM (1979) *Victorian Social Medicine: the ideas and methods of William Farr.* Johns Hopkins University Press, London and Baltimore.
6   Higgs E (1996) The statistical big bang of 1911: ideology, technological innovation and the production of medical statistics. *Social History of Medicine.* **9**(3): 409–26.
7   Office of Population Censuses and Surveys (1990) *Registration: proposals for change.* Cmd 939. HMSO, London.
8   Wigglesworth JS (1980) Monitoring perinatal mortality. A pathophysiological approach. *Lancet.* **ii**(8196): 684–6.
9   Alberman E, Botting B, Blatchley N and Twidell A (1994) A new hierarchical classification of causes of infant death in England and Wales. *Archives of Disease in Childhood.* **70**: 403–9.
10 Alberman E, Blatchley N, Botting B *et al.* (1997) Medical causes on stillbirth certificates in England and Wales: distribution and results of hierarchical classifications tested by the Office for National Statistics. *British Journal of Obstetrics and Gynaecology.* **104**(9): 1043–9.
11 Confidential Enquiry into Stillbirths and Deaths in Infancy (2000) *7th*

Annual Report. Maternal and Child Health Research Consortium, London.

12   Department of Health, Welsh Office, Scottish Office Department of Health, Department of Health and Social Services, Northern Ireland (1998) *Why Mothers Die. Report on confidential enquiries into maternal deaths in the United Kingdom, 1994–1996.* The Stationery Office, London.

13   Office for National Statistics (1999) *The National Congenital Anomaly System. A guide for data suppliers.* Office for National Statistics, London.

14   Office of Population Censuses and Surveys (1995) *The OPCS Monitoring Scheme for Congenital Malformation: a review by a working group of the Registrar General's Medical Advisory Committee.* Occasional paper 43. OPCS, London.

15   Rigby MJ (1987) The national child health system. In: Macfarlane JA (ed) *Progress in Child Health, Vol. 3.* Churchill Livingstone, Edinburgh.

16   Rigby M (1998) Information in child health management. In: Rigby M, Ross EM and Begg NT (eds) *Management for Child Health Services.* Chapman and Hall Medical, London, pp. 122–141.

17   Rigby MJ and Nolder D (1994) Lessons from a child health system on opportunities and threats to quality from networked record systems. In: Roger-France F, Noothoven van Goor J and Staehr-Johansen K (eds) *Case-based Telematic Systems Towards Equity Health Care.* Studies in health technologies and informatics, Vol. 14. IOS Press, Amsterdam.

18   Welsh Office (1998) *Maternity Aspects of Child Health in Wales.* Third report. WHSCSA, Cardiff.

19   Parkes J, Dolk H and Hill N (1998) Does the Child Health Computing System adequately identify children with cerebral palsy? *Journal of Public Health Medicine.* 20(1): 102–4.

20   Johnson A and King R (1999) Can routine information systems be used to monitor serious disability? *Archives of Disease in Childhood.* 80: 63–6.

21   Nightingale F (1871) *Introductory Notes on Lying-in Institutions.* Longmans, Green, and Co., London.

22   Macfarlane AJ (1984) Trends in maternity care. In: Office of Population Censuses and Surveys, Department of Health and Social Security, Welsh Office. *Hospital In-patient Enquiry: maternity tables 1977–1981.* MB4 No. 19. HMSO, London.

23   Department of Health, Office of Population Censuses and Surveys (1988) *Hospital In-patient Enquiry: maternity tables 1982–1985, England and Wales.* MB4 No. 28. HMSO, London.

24 Steering Group on Health Services Information (1982) *First Report to the Secretary of State*. HMSO, London.
25 Steering Group on Health Services Information (1985) *Supplement to the First and Fourth Reports to the Secretary of State*. HMSO, London.
26 Department of Health (1997) *NHS maternity statistics, England: 1989–90 to 1994–95*. Statistical Bulletin 1997/98. Department of Health, London.
27 Cleary R, Beard RW, Coles J et al. (1994) The quality of routinely collected maternity data. *British Journal of Obstetrics and Gynaecology*. **101**: 1042–7.
28 Kenney N and Macfarlane AJ (1999) Maternity data in England: problems with data collection at a local level. *British Medical Journal*. **319**: 619–22.
29 Information and Statistics Division (1997) *Births in Scotland 1975–1995*. ISD, Edinburgh.
30 Department of Health, NHS Executive (1998) *Information for Health*. NHS Executive, Leeds.
31 National Information Management and Technology Board (1998) *Strategic Programme for Modernising Information Management and Technology in the NHS in Scotland*. Scottish Office, Edinburgh.
32 Welsh Office (1998) *Better Information, Better Health: information management and technology for health care and health improvement in Wales. A strategic framework 1998 to 2005*. Welsh Office, Cardiff.
33 NHS Information Authority (2000) *For the Record: defining values in maternity*. NHS Information Authority, Winchester. http://www.nhsia.nhs.uk/med
34 NHS Information Authority (1999) *NHS Numbers for Babies*. NHS Information Authority, Exeter. http://www.nhsia.nhs.uk/nn46

Contact addresses and websites

Office for National Statistics
1 Drummond Gate, London SW1V 2QQ
General enquiries: 020 7533 5888
Website: http://www.statistics.gov.uk/

Published tables and specific enquiries:
  Births and fertility: 01329 813758
Topic enquiries
  Abortions: 020 7533 5112
  Conceptions: 020 7533 5137
  Congenital anomalies: 020 7533 5641
  Infant and perinatal mortality: 020 7533 5205

StatBase website: http://www.statistics.gov.uk/statbase/mainmenu.asp

General Register Office for Scotland
Ladywell House, Ladywell Road, Edinburgh EH12 7TF
Tel: 0131 314 4254
Website: http://www.gro-scotland.gov.uk

General Register Office for Northern Ireland
McAuley House, 2–14 Castle Street, Belfast BT1 1SA
Tel: 028 90 252031/2
Website: http://www.nisra.gov.uk/gro/

Department of Health
Statistical bulletins and most other publications are available from:
Department of Health, PO Box 777, London SE1 6XH
Tel: 0541 555 455
Fax: 01623 724524
Website: http://www.doh.gov.uk/

Branch SD2, Hospital and community health services statistics
Skipton House, 80 London Road, London SE1 6LW
Maternity statistics: 020 7972 5533

National Assembly for Wales, formerly the Welsh Office
Health statistics: 029 20 825080
Statistical publications:
Publications Unit, Statistical Directorate 5, National Assembly for Wales,
Cathay's Park, Cardiff CF10 3NQ
E-mail: statswales@gtnet.gov.uk

Information and Statistics Division, Common Services Agency of the NHS in Scotland
Trinity Park House, South Trinity Road, Edinburgh EH5 3SQ
Tel: 0131 552 6255
Website: http://www.show.scot.nhs.uk/isd/index.htm

Department of Health, Social Services and Public Safety, formerly Department of Health and Social Services
Regional Information Branch, Annex 2, Castle Buildings, Stormont,
Belfast BT4 3UD
Tel: 028 90 522800
Website: http://www.dhssni.gov.uk/

10 Cancer registries

Gillian Matthews

Introduction

This chapter describes the:

- system of cancer registration
- data collected, and its quality assurance
- standard outputs produced by cancer registries
- access to registry services
- opportunities for individual projects.

The system

What is cancer registration?

Cancer registration is the collection and classification of data on all cases of cancer occurring within a defined territory. It is essentially population based. However, within any catchment area, the cases recorded are both for those people resident in the area, and for those people who are non-resident but are treated within the area.

The international scene

Cancer registration is a world-wide process. The longest established cancer registries are in Europe and North America, but increasingly they are being developed in the emerging countries of Asia, Africa and South America.

Attempts to record comprehensive information on the incidence and distribution of cancer have been made as part of individual censuses and studies since the last century. But it was not until the late 1940s that momentum really got underway. In 1959 the World Health Organization (WHO) produced recommendations for the establishment of cancer registries, and, in 1965 the International Agency for Research on Cancer (IARC) was established as a specialist research centre of WHO. This in turn led to the formation in 1966 of the International Association of Cancer Registries.

Cancer registration in the UK

In the UK the development of cancer registries initially happened on a piecemeal basis. This has the inevitable consequence that the ability to portray time trends in the incidence of cancer varies in different parts of the country depending on the length of operation of the local databases. It was not until 1962 that all regions in England and Wales were incorporated into a comprehensive national cancer registration scheme. Cancer registration in Scotland evolved from a scheme similar to that in England and Wales.

While much good work, collecting and analysing data, has taken place through the second half of the twentieth century, the present era was ushered in by four Department of Health (DoH) circulars:

- EL(95)31 *Future Regional Public Health Role* explained arrangements for the purchasing of cancer registration and set out health authority responsibilities for a minimum level of service which they were required to secure.[1]

- EL(95)51 *A Policy Framework for Commissioning Cancer Services* (the Calman-Hine report), based on the work of the Expert Advisory Group on Cancer, emphasised the role of cancer registration data in the development of clinical cancer services. The report advocates concentration of expertise so that specialised treatment is available for different types of cancer.[2]

- EL(96)7 *Core Contract for Purchasing Cancer Registration* provided a model contract specification for use by purchasers in the NHS internal market and included a required national minimum dataset.[3]

- EL(96)15 *Implementing the Cancer Policy Framework*.[4]

Registry functions

NHS systems continue to change; first with the advent and now with abandonment of the NHS internal market. But the basic purposes and tasks involved in cancer registration remain the same.

NHS cancer registration tasks listed in the circular (EL(96)7) are:

- collection of complete, accurate and timely information
- provision of accurate and timely data for the Office of National Statistics (ONS) and to IARC in line with the minimum dataset

- dissemination of accurate and timely data for the compilation of national and international statistics
- undertaking research and development using registry data
- preparation of reports and educational material.

National policy on cancer registration in the NHS is overseen by the DoH Advisory Committee on Cancer Registration (ACCR). The current position is that continuing changes in NHS regional structures have a knock-on effect over the distribution and catchment of cancer registries. In 1999, NHS regions in London and Southern England were realigned with the creation of a London region and consequential changes in the NHS boundaries in the shire counties. Discussions are taking place as to the optimal configuration of the registry network in the affected regions, but decisions are not expected to be implemented until 2000/01.

At the same time the ACCR has initiated a review of organisational models for cancer registries. Again this may come to fruition in the year 2000.

At present there are nine English registries, and one each in Scotland, Wales and Northern Ireland. They are listed in Annex 1. The size of catchments relating to each registry varies significantly. The smallest serves a population of 1.7 million. The largest, Thames Cancer Registry (TCR), holds a database on the 13.8 million population of Greater London and the home counties; and size has implications for the operational systems used. A number of examples in this chapter are drawn from the work of TCR.

All the registries are members of the United Kingdom Association of Cancer Registries (UKACR). This is a professional association which sets service standards and fosters communication between registries.

In addition to the main registries there are certain specialist tumour registries with whom cancer registries exchange data. For example, there is the National Registry of Childhood Tumours at Oxford.

The data

Confidentiality and data protection

The primary source of data on which cancer registration is based is the patient's clinical case notes. This holds true whether the information is derived from hospital departments, primary or community care or the private sector.

Use of this information is a highly sensitive matter. This is recognised in *The Patients' Charter and You*, 1995,[5] which states categorically that 'everyone working for the NHS is under a legal duty to keep records confidential'.

In 1996 the DoH published guidance on *The Protection and Use of Patient Information.*[6] This document covers a broad field, but it is relevant to cancer registration in a number of respects:

- health professionals have an ethical duty of confidence in respect of patient personal information
- there is a need for patients to be fully informed of uses to which such information may be put
- personal data relating to living patients held on a computer system were subject to the Data Protection Act, 1984,[7] and are now subject to the Data Protection Act, 1998.[8] The 1998 Act implements the European Directive on the protection of individuals with regard to the processing of personal data, and on the free movement of personal data.[9] This EC Directive was adopted in 1995 and reinforces the NHS' own standards and obligations
- wherever possible personal information should be anonymised
- aggregated information may properly be used in
  - monitoring and protecting public health
  - managing and planning NHS services
  - clinical audit
  - medical or health service research
- management and staff at all levels are responsible for the physical security of the data, whether stored in manual records or on computer. Precise details are set out in a succession of documents issued by the NHS Executive, namely:
  - *Information Systems Security: top level policy for the NHS* (1992)[10]
  - EL(95)108 re. *The Protection of Information on the NHS Net*[11]
  - NHSE's *Security Reference Manual* (1996)[12]
- research proposals involving access to patient records require clearance by the relevant Local Research Ethics Committee.

Anyone planning to use registry data and who is not familiar with the processes involved would do well to read the DoH detailed guidance on the protection of patient information with thought and care.

The Data Protection Registrar also issues Guidelines (3rd Series, 1994)[13] listing eight principles which apply to holding and use of personal information embodied in the Data Protection Act, 1984. All cancer registries are required to be registered under the Data Protection Act.

Definition of cancers

EL(96)7 instructs registries to record 'all cases of those cancers included in the Annual Reference Volume of Cancer Registrations produced by ONS', leaving only a decision in respect of non-melanoma skin cancers to local discretion. Practice will vary marginally between registries. The Thames Cancer Registry (TCR), in its 1997 Annual Report,[14] specified its policy to register all invasive, in situ and borderline malignancies (except basal cell skin cancers). These correspond to ICD10 codes C00–C97, D00–D09, D37–D48. With a few listed exceptions, the benign neoplasms are not registered. In parallel with ICD10 TCR use ICD0 (oncology) which is specially adapted for neoplasms and includes classification coding for morphology and behaviour.

Minimum dataset

EL(96)7 sets out the minimum dataset of 22 items required for all inpatient and day cases. Additionally there are nine optional items suggested, and which most registries collect. Use of the material for a succession of projects creates a tendency to add ever more items on to the system. If unchecked this growth adds to the cost and slows down data processing. At TCR the use of all the historic data items was reviewed in 1997. This led to a reduction in the number of items collected. The current registration form (CRF3) adopted by TCR is shown in Annex 2.

TCR is working through a period of change with a view to collecting and transmitting data from cancer centres to the database electronically. The data items on this form will be collected whatever method of data transmission is used. However, there are difficulties in collecting some of this information using existing NHS trust IT systems, e.g. information in relation to clinical staging. The user of registry data should check that the dataset of any registry they approach meets their particular needs.

Data sources

Figure 10.1 illustrates the data sources and the flow of data between organisations. While the prime source of data is from a patient's case notes, death certificates from the ONS provide fall-back information which is recorded on the database. Currently NHS hospital trusts provide the bulk of the data. To complete the picture information is needed from hospices, the private sector, and from primary care.

Different registries vary as to the extent to which these further sources are included in their database. It is likely that the rapidly increased use of information technology within general practices and the demands of primary care service commissioning will bring added impetus to the collection of community data.

Data processing

Historically data have been retrieved manually by registry employees outposted in hospitals. In the Trent Region and Northern Ireland electronic systems are used. Some other registries, such as TCR, are currently engaged in changing over to electronic processing where hospital systems make this feasible.

Increasingly hospitals are developing their own internal clinical data systems. The ideal arrangement is for cancer registration data to fall out as a by-product of the trust's regular systems. This will ultimately improve the efficiency of both hospital and registry processes. However, the wide variation which exists between different trust information systems makes the present reality some way off from achieving the ideal.

Responsibility for the provision of data rests with the trust and its clinical staff. Different registries have developed a variety of mechanisms to raise the awareness and understanding of hospital consultants, because much of the quality of the exercise stands or falls on the basis of their initiatives in supplying source data.

Data quality

Registration performance targets

Interim and ultimate national targets were set out in EL(96)7. These address:

- levels of ascertainment
- completeness and accuracy of data on each registered case

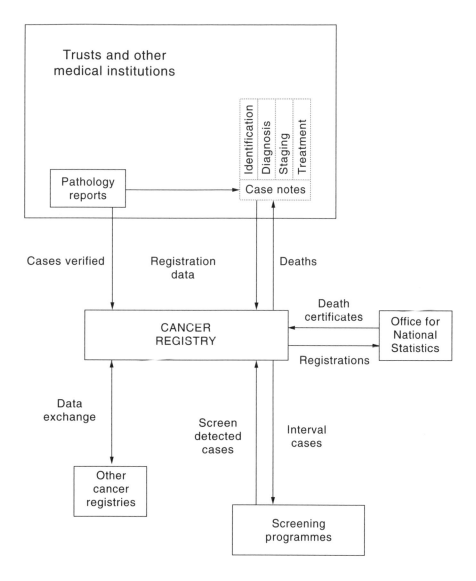

Figure 10.1 Cancer registration data sources.

- validity checks incorporated in registries' computer systems
- timeliness of registration from the date of original diagnosis
- reliability.

Detailed targets to which registries should aspire in 1999/2000 include:

- proportion of cases registered by death certificate only (DCO) – 2%

- coverage (compared with clinical and pathology source material) – 95%
- completeness, assessed by random case note checks (with NO transcription coding errors) – 95%
- tumour staging in respect of named key cancer sites (breast, cervix, and surgically treated colorectal and melanoma) – 80%
- timeliness – registration to be completed and entered on the database within a year of the initial diagnosis – 95%.

Success in achieving these targets has varied between different registries. Considerable management effort has been directed towards remedying historical deficiencies. Users of registry data need to make an assessment as to whether the material they seek is of sufficiently high quality for their specific purposes. They can do this by checking with the registries themselves, and these are listed in Annex 1. The formal reports of registries publish details on their performance, and this information can be cross-checked by contacting the ONS.

Validation of data

Tests are built into internal systems at the registries to ensure the accuracy and consistency of the data held. These include:

- format checks on incoming data, checking that the entries are correct and in the form required by the system
- code checks to see if the codes entered are valid, e.g. postcode, code for ethnic origin, hospital and consultant codes
- cross-validations to ensure consistency between data items, e.g. all patients registered with prostate cancer must be male
- specific checking of material received on magnetic media, e.g. to identify cases which require manual resolution; to link cases attending a series of hospitals or cancer centres.

Access

Access to cancer registration data

Data is collected in order that it may be used. Appropriate NHS staff may therefore ask registries for information required for NHS purposes as defined in the DoH Guidance (1996).[6] Bona fide researchers need to submit satisfactory protocols and give guarantees of meeting registry confidentiality requirements. Patients also have right of access to their personal details recorded on the database.

Registries supply data in a range of ways: in regular reports; in cancer fact sheets; on diskette; on the World Wide Web. A capability for direct access to data is being explored in some registries such as the Yorkshire and Northern Registry, enabling clients to carry out further analyses themselves.

Personal contact with either the director or information manager of a registry will lead to appropriate information being made available. An initial telephone call should be followed by a request in writing, which should cover:

- the purpose of the request
- how the information will be used
- type of analysis sought
- time period and geographical area to be covered
- types of cancer by ICD code
- user's deadlines.

This enables the registry to determine priorities between requests (in fairness to all users) and ensure the user receives the precise product needed.

Regular data exchange between the registry and other named organisations is an NHS requirement, e.g. with screening pro-grammes, ONS and IACR. Details of such exchanges are subject to negotiation between the organisations concerned.

Who uses registry data?

The main groups of people who approach registries seeking information are:

- health authorities
- NHS trusts, and individual clinicians
- genetic counsellors
- DoH, the NHSE, and in providing responses to parliamentary questions
- academic researchers (both UK and overseas)
- health charities
- press/media.

Requests from such users are in addition to data regularly provided on the basis of agreed data exchange as described above.

Registries are required to produce regular reports derived from their database relating to the population they serve. These reports are public documents and are widely available. The majority of individual requests are seeking descriptive, outcome or trend data. Because of the patient-specific linkage of hospital episode data which is incorporated in a registration, registries are also capable of providing patient flow data. This is difficult to obtain from standard HES data and is particularly needed by managers developing tertiary hospital services. Requests from the media would specifically need to be addressed to a registry's director.

The rest of this chapter now takes a more detailed look at the range of purposes for which cancer registration data are used.

Using cancer registry information

The reasons for which cancer registry information is sought vary according to the responsibilities and interests of the user. The following examples are not exhaustive but cover the main areas to which cancer registration can make a substantial contribution.

Health authorities

Health authorities and cancer registries share a common interest in a defined population base. Malignant disease creates a major burden of care for health authorities. Demographic changes in the age profile of the population imply a rising need. This has been emphasised by the priority given to the implementation of the Calman–Hine report[2] on cancer services and its recommended service model.

Health authorities have key duties to:

- assess service need
- commission hospital and some community services
- monitor performance in the trusts who provide their chosen service.

All these tasks require a statistical base so that need can be quantified and analysed, agreements reached with service providers, and both service performance and clinical outcome audited.

Health authorities may wish to commission special projects to meet particular local needs. Though the routine data available from and published by cancer registries will meet most of their requirements, they may want rates of malignant disease overall as well as details in respect of different types of tumour. They will also be interested in comparing their incidence rates as well as clinical outcomes with national standards and with their neighbouring or comparable authorities.

A standard package for a health authority is likely to cover:

- case numbers, crude rate and age-standardised rate
- crude rate by age and sex
- prevalence by age group
- trends in incidence rates
- treatment modality (radiotherapy, surgery, chemotherapy)
- referral patterns
- trends in 5-year survival rates.

Some registries will also be able to offer a mapping facility.

Where the basic figures illustrate significant or unusual differences from the national pattern, a health authority may well work with the registry and perhaps commission specific analyses. A helpful example of such a project is the Oxford Cancer Information Unit's 1995 report *Targeting Melanoma*[15] which is based on analyses of Oxford Cancer Registry data.

Health authorities will also be interested in outcome measures which reflect on the effectiveness of cancer screening programmes offered to their population.

Any report prepared by the registry should be accompanied by a statement describing any quality problems which may be affecting the information supplied and its interpretation.

Service assessment

In recent years there has been much anxiety expressed by the public over differences in the clinical quality of service available depending on where you live. The publication of hospital league tables is a sensitive subject. Commissioning of cancer registry services is currently undertaken by nominated lead purchasers on behalf of all the health authorities who make up the catchment served. The lead authorities reach service agreements with the registry and will look for information on trust performance in supplying the required case note data to the registry. However, information on clinical outcome would be regarded by the registry as appropriate in the first instance for hospital trusts; a health authority exploring the clinical quality of services would need to approach a trust directly.

Primary care groups

These have existed in shadow form during 1998, and on 1 April 1999 were created as sub-committees of health authorities. As their skills in meeting local service needs develop they may progress to become free-standing trusts. Their initial focus is on the provision of an effective and full range of primary care services. They also work with health authorities in commissioning secondary hospital services. They represent catchments of around 100 000 population and network with local authorities and other service organisations. In due course one can envisage PCGs seeking information to help them assess local needs in respect of continuing and terminal care cancer services as well as appraising secondary hospital services.

NHS hospital trusts

The sophistication of internal hospital information systems (HIS) varies widely in respect of both activity data and clinical databases. Their ability to provide cancer registration data automatically and electronically varies considerably, and work is continuing on this in some parts of the country. At the same time trust need for registry outputs is steadily increasing.

Trusts are interested in attracting patients and marketing trust services; in developing cost-effective models of care; in monitoring their own performance; and in clinical audit. The emphasis on clinical governance and trust accountability[16] for the quality of their clinical care will lead to greater trust interest in cancer data.

While the population-based figures that health authorities seek may be a helpful background for a trust developing its service, and patient flow data will describe the historic picture, it is in the area of audit that registry data have a most notable part to play. For this trusts will be looking for up-to-date data.

In response to trust requests a registry can provide:

- service performance dataset against a background of anonymised aggregated multi-trust data
- clinical performance data such as tumour staging and historical verification of malignant disease

- cancer deaths by consultant and clinical unit
- detailed clinical audit (*see* below).

Further trust-specific information can be arranged in response to individual requests.

Clinical audit

The public increasingly wishes to be kept informed on the quality of care it can expect to receive. The demand is for openness. Nonetheless, it is understandable that the most successful exploration of clinical outcome standards is usually carried out by cooperation between the professional staff concerned and NHS management. Examples in the London area have all been clinician based and, indeed, clinician led.

Thus a continuing prospective audit of the treatment of breast cancer in North Thames hospitals is steered by a clinical group and receives cancer registry data analysed against hospital characteristics.[17]

In South Thames an initiative instigated by the Haematology Specialist Committee has taken the process a stage further. TCR has been commissioned by the haematologists jointly to run their Haematology Register with them.[18] This has led to constructive and joint working between the registry and the clinicians, agreement on the dataset to be used and a range of products which enable the haematologists to examine the service they offer. At the same time the work involved also improves the quality of input to the registry's database.

The ability to set up multi–trust systems in this way using cancer registry experience and skills is particularly useful in smaller clinical specialties where the volume of work passing through a single trust may be insufficient to provide a balanced view on their individual service.

This is a growth area. The process starts with clinical specialists seeing the benefits to be derived from a degree of standardisation in their services. This leads to the development of a common dataset, such as that recently produced by the Royal College of Pathologists covering histopathology. Thereafter they can seek a contribution from cancer registration in a range of ways – from simple listing of appropriate cases for review, to the management of clinical audit as instanced by the South Thames haematologists.

National viewpoint

The DoH and NHSE have a particular interest in the output of cancer registries. This is expressed in a number of ways.

- *Incorporation of cancer data in the work and outputs of the ONS.* This is secured by regular data transfer from registries to the ONS.

- *Monitoring service performance.* For example, drawing on the dataset which tracks a patient's clinical pathway, a registry can provide information on time intervals between referral, diagnosis and treatment. This facility has been used in the DoH 1998 Cancer Waiting Times Audit (HSE 1998/014)[19,20] and HSC 1998/065 *The New NHS: modern, dependable*[21] identifies a variety of contributions cancer registration can make in monitoring service performance.

- *Audit of service policy.* Depending on the timescale taken to reshape clinical services along the lines recommended in the Calman-Hine report,[2] registries will soon be in a position to provide information on the degree of specialisation available for the treatment of named cancers, and to compare patient flows before and after the implementation of cancer services and units. Information on clinical outcomes will take longer – but in due course should be apparent.

- The government's Health Improvement Programme outlined in *The New NHS: modern, dependable* includes a *National Contract on Cancer.* The identification of cancer as one of the four clinical areas given priority is because of the high prevalence of malignant disease and the scope for improvement in its diagnosis, care and outcomes. It will be part of the wider Cancer Information Strategy, which the DoH is developing to underpin the priority it is giving to the provision of cancer services. An up-to-date position on this initiative can be obtained from the NHS Information Authority website at www.cancer.nhsia.nhs.uk. Cancer registration data will be critical to the monitoring and assessment of the national contract.

- *Audit of cancer screening programmes.* Cancer registries in the first instance contribute to the quality control of screening programmes, such as that for breast cancer, by regular data exchange with screening units. Registries can identify cases which arise between mammography examinations, and these data are passed to the screening programme.

In the longer term both specific research studies and publication of trends in population-based incidence rates will illustrate the impact of national cancer screening programmes. Due allowance needs to be made for confounding variables such as age and social class. Nonetheless, at macro-policy level it should be possible to demonstrate results over time in terms of lowered incidence and prevalence rates.

Research

The opportunities for research using cancer registry data are extensive and varied. They may be constrained by resources but are only limited by the capacity to formulate relevant hypotheses and devise research protocols. Formal ethical approval is an essential prerequisite.

The majority of studies carried out consist of epidemiological analyses:

- describing an affected population – incidence, prevalence, mortality
- exploring correlation with variables that may be causative
- identifying relative risk of contracting named cancers
- time trends
- mapping
- survival and other outcomes.

In addition research can be carried out into cancer registration methodology. Multicentre and multinational studies can illuminate differences in incidence and outcomes. The Eurocare Study,[22] published in 1995, demonstrated significant differences in 5-year survival from breast cancer experienced in 12 European countries. Occupational risks can be identified. The association of mesothelioma with exposure to asbestos is a well-known example.

A bona fide researcher wishing to use cancer registry data will start by making an informal approach, seeking a preliminary exploration of the concept and feasibility with the director or other appropriate registry staff. Before funding is sought for a project the researcher will need to:

- devise a protocol (including any pilot exercise)
- seek peer review of the protocol
- obtain ethical approval

- guarantee adherence to the registry's confidentiality conditions
- identify the data and possible analyses sought
- agree a work programme.

Initial attention to setting up a research project in a correct way is not only essential to the probity and quality of the research, but in a practical sense should avoid problems at a late stage in the exercise.

While the majority of historic studies have been led by medically or scientifically qualified researchers there is nothing to prevent professional workers in other disciplines from carrying out research based on registration data. One can envisage the range of researchers widening as possibilities for studying cancer patients' quality of life are developed.

Conclusion

Cancer registration:

- provides a service with far-reaching implications
- technology and methods are being reviewed and modernised
- has a major contribution to make in the modern NHS – particularly as part of clinical and service audit
- data are only a phone call away.

References

1 NHS Executive (1995) *Future Regional Public Health Role*. Executive Letter EL(95)31. NHSE, Leeds.
2 NHS Executive (1995) *A Policy Framework for Commissioning Cancer Services: Calman-Hine report*. Executive Letter EL(95)51. NHSE, Leeds.
3 NHS Executive (1996) *Core Contract for Purchasing Cancer Registration*. Executive Letter EL(96)7. NHSE, Leeds.
4 NHS Executive (1996) *Implementing the Cancer Policy Framework*. Executive Letter EL(96)15. NHSE, Leeds.
5 NHS Executive (1995) *The Patients' Charter and You*. Department of Health, London.
6 Department of Health (1996) *The Protection and Use of Patient Information*. Department of Health, London.
7 Data Protection Act 1984. HMSO, London.
8 Data Protection Act 1998. HMSO, London.
9 EC Directive on Data Protection. European Directive 95/46/EC.

10   NHS Executive (1992) *Information Systems Security: top level policy for the NHS.* NHS Management Executive, Leeds.

11   NHS Executive (1995) *The Protection of Information on the NHS Net.* Executive Letter EL(95)108. NHSE, Leeds.

12   NHS Executive (1996) *Security Reference Manual.* NHSE, Leeds.

13   Data Protection Registrar (1994) *The Guidelines (3rd Series).* Data Protection Registrar, London.

14   Thames Cancer Registry (1997) *Cancer in South East England 1996.* Thames Cancer Registry, London.

15   Oxford Cancer Intelligence Unit (1995) *Targeting Melanoma: a priority for the Health of the Nation.* Oxford Cancer Intelligence Unit, Oxford.

16   Department of Health (1998) *A First Class Service: quality in the new NHS.* Department of Health, London.

17   Bell J and Ma M (1997) *Prospective Audit of Breast Cancer.* Thames Cancer Registry, London.

18   Thames Cancer Registry/Haematology Specialist Committee (1998) *South Thames Haematology Register.* Thames Cancer Registry, London.

19   NHS Executive (1998) *Cancer Waiting Times Audit.* Health Service Circular HSC 1998/014. NHSE, Leeds.

20   NHS Executive (1998) *Cancer Waiting Times Audit: methodology and funding.* Health Service Circular HSC 1998/046. NHSE, Leeds.

21   Department of Health (1997) *The New NHS: modern, dependable.* Cmd 3807. The Stationery Office, London.

22   Eurocare (1995) *Breast Cancer in Europe.* Eurocare Coordinating Centre, Lombardy Cancer Registration, Divisione di Epidemiologica, Instituto Nationale Tumori, Via Venezian 1.20133, Milano, Italy.

Annex 1   United Kingdom Cancer Registries

Registry	*Director's telephone no.*
East Anglian Cancer Registry Addenbrooke's Hospital Hills Road Cambridge CB2 2QQ	01223 330318
Merseyside and Cheshire Cancer Registry 2nd Floor, Muspratt Building The University of Liverpool Liverpool L69 3BX	0151 794 5690
North Western Cancer Registry Centre for Cancer Epidemiology Christie Hospital NHS Trust Kinnaird Road Withington Manchester M20 9QL	0161 446 3575
Northern and Yorkshire Cancer Registry and Information Service Arthington House Cookridge Hospital Leeds LS16 6QB	0113 292 4163
Oxford Cancer Intelligence Unit Oxfordshire Health Old Road Headington Oxford OX3 7LF	01865 226742
South and West Cancer Intelligence Unit (Bristol) Grosvenor House 149 Whiteladies Road Bristol BS8 2RA	0117 970 6474
South and West Cancer Intelligence Unit (Winchester) Highcroft Romsey Road Winchester SO22 5DH	01962 863511

Thames Cancer Registry   020 7378 7688
1st Floor, Capital House
Weston Street
London SE1 3QD

Trent Cancer Registry   0114 226 5351
Floor 6, Weston Park Hospital NHS Trust
Whitham Road
Sheffield S10 2SJ

West Midlands Cancer Intelligence Unit   0121 414 7711
The Public Health Building
University of Birmingham
Birmingham B15 2TT

Northern Ireland Cancer Registry   01232 263136
Department of Epidemiology & Public Health
Queen's University of Belfast
Mulhouse Building
Institute of Clinical Science
Grosvenor Road
Belfast BT12 6BT

National Health Service in Scotland   0131 551 8562
Information and Statistics Division
Trinity Park House
South Trinity Road
Edinburgh EH5 2SQ

Wales Cancer Intelligence and Surveillance   01222 373500
    Unit
14 Cathedral Road
Cardiff CF1 9JL

Annex 2

Thames Cancer Registry - Capital House Weston Street London SE1 3QD Tel: 0171 378 7688 **CRF3**

Old TCR number |___|___|___|___|___|___|___| TCR number |___|___|___|___|___|___|___|

Identification details

Surname _____	Date of birth |___|___|___|___|___|___|
Forename(s) _____	Maiden name _____

	Address at diagnosis	**Other address**	
			Place of birth _____
Street	_____	_____	Ethnic origin _____
Town	_____	_____	NHS No. |_____|
County	_____	_____	Sex: M F I X |___|
Country	_____	_____	Marital status M S W D P C X |___|
Postcode |___|___|___|___| |___|___|___|___|		Occupation

GP practice _____   GP code |_____|

Date GP referral letter written |___|___|___|___|___|___| Date GP referral letter received |___|___|___|___|___|___|

Basis of diagnosis	CL = Clinical	XR = XRay	SC = Scan	EX = Exploratory	MA = Marker
	CY = Cytology	HE = Haematology	HM = Hist Mets	HI = Histology	PM = Post mortem
	DC = Death cert.	XX = Not known			|___|

Path report seen? Y *Or* N |___|

Date of diagnosis |___|___|___|___|___|___|

Morphology of 1°

Behaviour of 1°	0 = Benign	1 = Borderline	2 = In situ	3 = Invasive	X = Not known |___|

Differentiation	1 = Well (G1)	2 = Moderate (G2)	3 = Poor (G3)	4 = Undiff/anaplastic	|___|
	5 = T cell	6 = B cell	7 = Null cell	X = Not stated	

Primary site   Side L R B N X |___|

Distant metastases? |___| Location of 2°

Clinical TNM (As stated in case notes)   T   N   M |___|___|___|

Path TNM (As stated in path. report)   PT   PN   PM |___|___|___|

Direct extension? |___|

Nodes sampled? |___| How many? |___|___|

Positive nodes? |___| How many? |___|___|

Tumour size (mm)	**Other malignancy?** Y *Or* N |___|
Stage/Grade _____	Site _____ Year |___|___|

Treatment details

Surgery Y ☐ N ☐

Date	Hospital	Consultant	Specialty	Operation

Radiotherapy Y ☐ N ☐

Date	Hospital	Consultant

Chemotherapy Y ☐ N ☐

Date	Hospital	Consultant

Hormone Y ☐ N ☐

Date	Hospital	Consultant

Notes

All hospitals visited

Date	Hospital	Case note No.	Refer for*

Refer for: D = date of birth P = path. report A = address G = grade/stage T = treatment S = side F = full registration

CRF3 Ver.4 12.11.98   R.O. |_____| Date |____|____|____|____|

11 Statistical data linkage

Colin Cryer

Introduction

Data linkage brings together data from two or more sources at the individual level. It is very frequently used when the data from one source do not satisfy our information needs. For example, in injury research we are interested in the association between the circumstances of an incident that led to an injury (e.g. details of the circumstances of a crash between a car and a motorcyclist), and the nature and severity of the injuries that occurred (e.g. for the motorcyclist, fracture of the thoracic spine [neck] with spinal cord involvement). This type of information can be helpful in identifying those factors that increase the probability of injury occurrence, and in identifying methods for:

- reducing the chances of an incident occurring
- reducing the severity of injury should an incident occur
- reducing the likelihood of death or disability as an outcome.

No one source of routinely collected data provides information both on the circumstances of the incident, and a good description of the type and severity of injuries that result. Data on circumstances are routinely available for some types of accidents (e.g. road, work, and fire-related) and data on outcomes are available in other data sources (e.g. hospital inpatient data). This gives the motivation to link data sources.

This chapter is concerned with those issues that we need to consider when linking together secondary data sources at the individual level with the aim of producing a richer database. As an illustration, I will use the linkage of police road traffic accident reports to the data that are collected when people are admitted to hospital. Although this is a very specific example, many of the points that I make are relevant to other areas. Other examples of data linkage are shown in Box 11.1.

One reason to focus attention on accidental injury is that accidents are an important cause of premature mortality and morbidity.[1] An interest in the prevention of accidental injury exists at both the governmental and local levels. Both the previous government's health strategy, *The Health of the Nation*,[2] and the present government's health strategy, *Saving Lives: our healthier nation*,[3] identified accidents as a priority area. This new health strategy, along with the White Paper *The New NHS*,[4] is promoting much activity at the local level through multi-agency health improvement programmes (HImPs). Many of these include a component for the reduction of the rate of accidental injuries.

In this chapter, I will answer the following questions:

- why are we interested in linking secondary data sources?
- for accident prevention and injury control, what data sources is it feasible to link?
- what data linkage methods can be used?
- what are the barriers to linking data sources?
- do the linked data satisfy our needs?

Each of these questions will be addressed in turn by each of the sections that follow. The chapter ends with the conclusion that there are a number of benefits associated with data linkage, but there is also a cost. The degree of benefit will depend upon the application, and an assessment needs to be made as to whether the benefit justifies the cost.

Box 11.1   Examples of data linkage using health-related data

- OPCS longitudinal study[5]
- Scottish record linkage system[6]
- Paediatric epidemiological research: birth data (e.g. birth records, midwife records) to morbidity and mortality data (e.g. hospital inpatient data)[7]
- Surveillance of occupational injury: work history (union membership files, medical insurance files) to injury data (e.g., worker's compensation records)[8]
- Child health surveillance for vulnerable groups: register of neonatal intensive care to the child health record[9]
- Aid to development and joint care planning: social services community care assessments to community health service data[10]
- Finnish national longitudinal health register for children: linkage of multiple data sources including birth, death, hospital discharge, intellectually disabled, cancer, and visual impairment registers[11]
- Determining first admissions in hospital inpatient data: linkage of hospital inpatient stays due to injury in a given year to subsequent stays[12]

Why data linkage?

Some of the reasons why we want good accident and injury data are listed in Box 11.2. To understand better the information needs within injury control, terms are described and a model of injury causation explained.

Box 11.2   The role of information in accident prevention and injury control

1   To describe the distribution of accidents and injuries
2   To identify who is getting injured, where, when and in what circumstances
3   To inform priority setting
4   To identify cause of accidents/injuries
5   To suggest methods of prevention
6   To identify the long-term effect of accidents and injuries
7   To influence resource allocation
8   To monitor trends

Accidents are unintentional events which can lead to injury. One definition of injury is as follows:

> Injury is tissue damage resulting from either the acute transfer to individuals of one of five forms of physical energy (kinetic or mechanical, thermal, chemical, electrical, or radiation), or from the sudden interruption of normal energy patterns necessary to maintain life processes.[13]

Examples of the latter are drownings and frostbite.

A very useful aid to analysis, strategy identification, and planning is the Haddon matrix.[14] It is based on two dimensions. The first dimension acknowledges the epidemiological model of injury causation which involves the interaction between the host, the agent, the vehicles/vectors of injury, and the environment. These terms, as they apply to injury epidemiology, are explained in Box 11.3. The second dimension recognises that injury events can be considered in

---

Box 11.3   Terminology

Host	= the injured person
Agent	= the various forms of energy which when transferred to the host at sufficiently high levels result in injury (e.g. thermal energy)
Vehicles/vectors	= objects or living things that convey the damaging energy (e.g. hot water)
Environment	= social and physical surroundings in which the event occurs

---

three stages: the pre-event, the event, and the post-event phases. This matrix can be used as an aid to identify systematically:

- pre-event factors – that influence the occurrence of the event (the accident)
- event factors – that affect the likelihood of injury given that an event has occurred, and
- post-event factors – that affect the long-term outcome of the injury (e.g. disability and death).

An example of the Haddon matrix applied to falls in older people is shown in Table 11.1.

Table 11.1 Selected risk factors for falls and their sequelae in older people

	Human	Vehicle/vector	Social environment	Physical environment
Pre-event	Poor sight	Own momentum	Living alone; no help or support	Uneven stair heights
Event	Osteoporosis (brittle bones)	Own momentum	Padded hip protectors not on prescription	Lack of stair rails
Post-event	Rehabilitation to return function to pre-fall levels		No help to get up; long lie	No call alarm button to summon help

We wish to access data that are sufficient to satisfy the information requirements listed in Box 11.2. In order to do this, we would like our data sources to include data on the accident characteristics, on the personal characteristics of the injured person, and on the consequences of the accident and the injury.[15]

Relevant data sources which are readily available to the NHS are the registrations of deaths and hospital inpatient data (*see* Chapters 2 and 4). These data sources provide good information on the consequences of accidents, but contain limited data on where the event occurred, and how it occurred. Data sources from other agencies tend to have a wealth of information on the circumstances of the accident, but have limited information on the consequences.

Linkage of these two types of data source is a potential route to enhancing the quality of information available for accident prevention and injury control. This sentiment is echoed by the Public Health Information Strategy Report[16] in which it is stated:

If the basic information on an accident/person involved in an accident was comparable or could be linked between each source, the overlaps in scope would provide means for checking the coverage/completeness achieved within each source, as well as a means of aggregating all the different sets of information on any one accident. Collectively, more information is available than is contained in any one source.

The choice of data sources to link

A reasonably comprehensive and informative review of data sources was produced by the Public Health Information Strategy Group.[15] They identified a number of the major sources of routinely collected data relevant to accident/injury prevention, and these are listed in Box 11.4.

Box 11.4 Main accident/injury sources

Weaker on circumstance
- A&E department data
- Ambulance records
- GP data
- Hospital inpatient data
- Coroner's records
- Mortality statistics (ONS)
- Health Survey for England – HSFE (SCPR)
- General Household Survey – GHS (ONS)

Stronger on circumstance
- Home and leisure accident statistics – HASS/LASS (DTI)
- Fire statistics (Home Office)
- Road traffic accident reports (DETR)
- Health and Safety statistics (HSE)

I will use linkage to hospital inpatient data to illustrate the points I wish to make in this chapter since inpatient records represent the most complete and highest quality health dataset in England. Additionally, injury that results in admission is a major cost to the individual, to society and to the NHS in terms of disability, loss of quality of life, and monetary cost.[17]

Only three data sources that are strong on the circumstances of injury are serious candidates for linkage to inpatient data at the local level. These are the road accident data (STATS19),[18] the Health and Safety Executive's (HSE) database of work-related injury and dangerous occurrences (the RIDDOR database),[19,20] and fire statistics collated by the Home Office.

STATS19 collects a great deal of information on the circumstances of an accident for cases injured on the road. Many of these casualties are admitted to hospital. This large number of cases makes an investigation of linkage worthwhile, particularly since STATS19 has very limited information on the nature of the injuries and subsequent outcomes. There are a number of variables which could be used for linkage that are similar in the STATS19 and inpatient systems: age, sex, date of accident/admission, and type of road user. Additionally, names and addresses are available within the police's paper records if these are needed for linkage.

The HSE's RIDDOR system includes data on work-related injuries which result in an absence from work for more than three days, and reportable dangerous occurrences. There are significant practical barriers to using these data for data linkage, however. There is gross under-reporting of events to the HSE[21] and so only a proportion of eligible cases will be available for matching. Additionally, since the hospital system does not record whether a case is work related or not, there will be difficulties in identifying relevant cases for matching from the inpatient data. The provision of personal data by the HSE to third parties would require informed consent from the casualty, which could reduce substantially the number of cases available for matching.

For the fire statistics, although there are a relatively small number of cases which are admitted to hospital compared with these other sources, the numbers may be sufficient to justify linkage. Some detailed information on the circumstances of the injury are recorded. Subject to satisfying data protection and Home Office requirements, these fire statistics are available for research purposes.

The above suggests that any one of these three sources could, in theory, be considered for linkage; however, it also suggests a higher likelihood of benefit and of success when linking STATS19 to inpatient data. This is the example I will use during the rest of this chapter.

Work commissioned by the Department of Health[15] identified a number of data items that are required for an accident database (shown in Table 11.2). It can be seen from this table that STATS19 data complement that available from inpatient systems. Within a linked database the majority of data items recommended by this

Table 11.2 Accident information requirements

Structure	Items	STATS19	Hospital inpatient data
Accident characteristics	Place of occurrence	✓	
	Geographic identifier of location	✓	
	Type	✓	✓
	Circumstances	✓	
Personal characteristics	Age and sex	✓	✓
	Area of residence		✓
	Socio-economic		?✓
	Ethnic group		✓
	Activity	✓	
	Predisposing factors	?	
Consequences	Nature of injury		✓
	Severity of injury	?	?✓
	Health service impact		✓
	Outcome	?	?

Key: ✓ = Recorded on the database
?✓ = Indicator can be generated from the database
? = Only limited information available
<blank> = No information available

report[15] would be available. Consequently, the expectation was that such a linked database would give a much more powerful base for injury control.

Choosing the data linkage method

Data linkage methods range from those where the link is made by manual searching to those that are solely electronically based. In general, manual linkage is more expensive and time consuming; however, its use can result in better linkage rates. On the other hand, automatic methods are generally cheaper and less time consuming, but they can lead to much poorer linkage rates. These two extremes will be considered below.

Automatic methods can be either deterministic or probabilistic. The theory of probabilistic record linkage can be found elsewhere.[22,23] In synopsis, combinations of variables (e.g. age, sex, type of road user, date of accident/admission) are compared from the two files for every possible pair of records, giving a separate score to each field based on matches or mismatches. The scores are combined across the relevant variables for a pair of records, to give the relative likelihood that the records belong to the same person. A rule can be set up such that records are linked if this likelihood exceeds some specified threshold.

One manual and two automatic approaches to deterministic record linkage are described below for linking inpatient data to STATS19 records. The fields used for linkage in the manual and automatic methods are shown in Box 11.5.

Box 11.5 Linkage fields used when linking hospital inpatient records to police road traffic accident data

Manual: Name; date of accident/admission
Validation fields: age; sex; type of road user
Automatic (1): Age; sex; type of road user; date of accident/admission
Automatic (2): Age (±5 years); sex; type of road user; date of accident/admission (same day or next day)

Manual linkage

In our work, the following procedure was followed.[24] A manual search of the police accident registers (books) was carried out for names and dates of accidents that approximately matched the names and dates of admission on each of the hospital records. If a match was identified, the accident reference number was obtained from the police register and added to the electronic hospital inpatient record. These records were then linked to the relevant STATS19 records using the accident reference number as the linking variable. All the links, and any multiple matches, were checked by comparing the information on age, sex, type of road user, and date of accident/admission between the two electronic databases. For 21% of those cases which were linked, the match had to be confirmed through inspection of the individual police accident records (paper files), because of lack of correspondence on one or more of these variables. This process resulted in 85% of the cases from one of the pilot hospitals being linked to the police data. This was slightly less than that achieved by Austin[25] who reported linkage rates of 89.9% by manually matching the two sets of records.

Automated data linkage

Strategies for automatic computer-based linkage were investigated by testing the situation where names and addresses are unknown.

This would be the case if only the electronic police data were used for linking. Two linkage methods were used and tested as follows.

1 Records were linked when there were exact matches on the variables of age, sex, date of admission/accident, and type of road user.

2 The above method was repeated but with tolerances, i.e. the date of admission could be up to 1 day after the date of the accident and still represent a match, and the recorded ages could be up to 5 years apart.

These methods were applied to the database of the cases for which a manual link between the hospital and STATS19 cases had been established, but with the links broken for this test. The results are shown in Table 11.3. These results are similar to those found by Nicholl,[26] but are inferior to those of Stone[27] applied to Scottish inpatient records, who both used similar approaches.

Table 11.3 Linkage performance when using automatic deterministic methods for those records previously linked using manual methods

	Cases linked (%)	Inaccurate links (%)	Multiple links (%)
Automatic (1)	52	0	0
Automatic (2)	81	1	7

We also attempted to link the hospital admission cases to the STATS19 database for all crashes which had occurred in the relevant geographic areas (including those that could not be linked using manual methods), but this resulted in an impracticably large number of duplicate matches being formed for both automatic methods.

On obtaining these results, it was decided, with our health authority and county council clients, that automatic matching without names and addresses was too problematic to consider for this application. The decision regarding what method is most efficient in other applications will be heavily dependent on the data sources being linked, the data they hold, the degree of overlap in the cases captured by each database, the accuracy of the data that is used for linking records, and the degree to which cases are uniquely determined by the linking variables.

Barriers

There are a number of potential practical, ethical, legal and administrative barriers to data linkage, which include those listed in Box 11.6, and which are described below.

Box 11.6   Potential barriers to record linkage

- Ethical
  - informed consent
  - confidentiality
- Data protection
  - confidentiality
  - fair obtaining
- Administrative
  - permission from data custodians
  - ethical approval
  - Data Protection registration
- Cost
- Time

Data linkage is not routinely carried out between NHS and non-NHS data sources, and so it is often regarded as a research activity. As such it requires ethical approval. If it is carried out in more than five centres, application needs to be made firstly to the relevant Multi-Centre Research Ethics Committee (MREC), and then to each of the local committees (LRECs). At least 3 months, and possibly as much as 6 months, should be planned for this process.

When seeking ethical approval for our study, there were a number of ethical issues raised. These included:

- whether or not informed consent is needed
- the potential for police access to confidential health data.

In regard to the latter, the chair of the MREC felt that it would be unacceptable in this country for the police to collect unselected accident data from NHS hospitals. This problem was overcome by ensuring that the hospital data remained confidential to the research team and kept about the researcher's person at all times, and through written assurance from the police that there would be no reason why anyone in the police station would require access to the data brought in by the researchers.

The argument made at the time against obtaining informed consent from each person whose records could potentially be linked was as follows. The data used in the study had already been collected by hospital staff and by police. Hospital data are collected to be used not only for patient care but also for statistical purposes. For this reason, the contract minimum dataset, which includes names and addresses,[28] is already made available to health authorities. Likewise, police road traffic accident reports are collected not only for evidence if a conviction is to be pursued, but also for statistical purposes to inform prevention, planning and evaluation. The project brought police data into the health authority for linkage, and I obtained confirmation from the Criminal Justice Department that this represented no problems for the purpose described using the methods outlined earlier in this chapter. Only aggregate information derived from the computerised hospital record and the police STATS19 record was generated by this project for the same purpose that health authorities already use this data, e.g. for planning. In their work, it would be extremely unusual for health authorities to seek informed consent from patients for this type of statistical analysis.

Although our registration under the Data Protection Act, at the time this work was carried out, covered the linkage of the STATS19 data to hospital inpatient records, there is some doubt whether an application now to the Data Protection Registrar would find favour. The changes to, and the interpretation of, the Act are such that this type of data linkage may not be acceptable in future without individual informed consent. Obviously, this would be a major barrier, since it would significantly increase the cost of linkage, and may substantially reduce the possible linkage rate.

In order to obtain names and addresses of people admitted to hospital, we had to approach each trust included in the study area. Initially, permission was sought and obtained from trust chief executives before a request for the data was made to the information manager within each trust. The elapsed time between seeking the relevant permission and the last of the trusts producing the extracts of hospital inpatient data was several months. The time involved was a function of the number of trusts approached; for our most recent work, which dealt with crashes that occurred across two counties, we approached 12 trusts. However, if this work were to become routine, then the time delays would be less. Between getting the appropriate ethical approval and obtaining all relevant data the time delays can be substantial. The cost, also, can be significant.

Does data linkage satisfy our needs?

The potential benefits of data linkage are listed in Box 11.7. These will be addressed in turn.

Box 11.7 Benefits of data linkage

- Enhance information (link circumstances to outcomes)
- Identify missing cases
- Identify biases in existing data systems
- Identify data inaccuracies

Increasing information available for injury prevention

Although all hospital cases could not be linked, for those that could, a more comprehensive data record was created than would be available otherwise. This additional data provided insight into what was causing the accidents that result in hospital admission, and so helped guide prevention. The additional information from hospital systems on the impact and severity of the injury enhanced STATS19 data and gave the facility to identify some of the circumstances that resulted in the most severe injuries, and which have the greatest impact on health service use.

Identifying missing cases

Eighty-five per cent of the injury cases, caused by road traffic accidents, from one of the pilot hospital's records were linked in our pilot. The failure to link the remaining 15% is likely to be due in most instances to cases which were admitted to hospital but which were not ascertained by the police. This problem of missing cases could be addressed in a number of ways, including modifying procedures for ascertainment of data or through inclusion of missing cases to enhance the police datasets used for analysis.

Identifying biases in existing data sources

The linkage rates were found to vary with type of road user (from best to worst): occupants of motor vehicles, motorcyclists, pedal cyclists, and pedestrians. The gradient in linkage rates between road users was likely to be due to differential reporting rates of accidents to the police. The proportion of unlinked cases also varied with age. Others' work has suggested that there were greater proportions of unlinked cases among those least seriously injured.[29] Use of the police data alone would, therefore, give a biased picture of the occurrence of road traffic accidents.

Identifying data inaccuracies

Identification of mismatches between STATS19 data and hospital inpatient data for particular fields can facilitate improvements in the data on both systems, and hence improve their usefulness.

Data linkage was used as a means to test for inaccurate data. The data on type of road user corresponded exactly. The date of accident corresponded with the date of admission in almost all cases. For sex, 9% of the cases differed. For age, 63% corresponded exactly, for 86% they were within 5 years of one another, but for 8% they differed by over 10 years. These results are consistent with other work. The weight of evidence suggests that the major inaccuracies in these variables are in the STATS19 rather than the hospital data. Both this study and others found that a large percentage of the cases were incorrectly classified by the police as 'slight' rather than 'serious' accidents. This field is influential in the analysis and planning by the County Council Highways and Transport Division (CCH&T), and so represents a major biasing factor. Correction of these known data errors in the STATS19 database would produce an immediate improvement to the data used by the CCH&T.

Conclusion

The previous description has indicated that for this application there are a number of definite benefits of data linkage. It allowed the CCH&T to quantify road traffic accident cases of which they were previously unaware, in their previous analysis of police road traffic accident reports, and to go some way to quantifying the magnitude of the under-reporting of accidents, and thus the potential bias, for different groups, e.g. by type of road user.

The CCH&T were made more aware of the inaccuracies in the police data. It was surprising that such a large number of cases had an incorrect sex recorded, and that the ages between the two data sources were so discrepant. Without correction for these errors, bias would result. It was less surprising that there were significant inaccuracies in the classification by the police of the severity of injury of the casualty. It must be very difficult for the police to accurately assess the severity of many injuries at the road-side.

Although these inaccuracies are understandable, they may be crucial in terms of the way in which the police data are used by the CCH&T department for accident prevention planning. When priority setting, those crashes that result in the most severe injury are given greatest weight by CCH&T, in the particular county being studied. The use of the crude and inaccurate severity coding within STATS19 could, therefore, be highly misleading. A major bonus of the linkage to hospital admission data was not only that it provided the ability to correct these severity coding inaccuracies, but it also provides potentially better severity measures based on diagnosis, length of stay, procedures used in hospital, ward of treatment, and discharge destination.

Potential benefits can result for any data linkage application. Data linkage will permit the identification of cases present in one data source that are absent in another, and thus give the opportunity to identify and correct for bias in the future. It will allow the accuracy of fields, which are common to both linked data sources, to be assessed. Further investigation will determine which values are accurate and which inaccurate. Once known, this again will permit biases to be identified and corrected in future. Finally, the availability of a much more comprehensive data record will almost certainly be beneficial. The degree of benefit will, however, be very dependent on the application.

Balanced against all of this is the often substantial cost of carrying out data linkage work. As often occurs with information applications, it is very difficult to quantify the benefits in such a way that will justify a substantial outlay in terms of cost and time. In our work, the results of the pilot showed the potential for major biases without data linkage which would mislead future planning. This was sufficient to persuade the health authority and the county council that future work in this area was likely to be cost-beneficial.

References

1 Cryer PC, Davidson L, Styles CP *et al.* (1996) Descriptive epidemiology of injury in the South East: identifying priorities for action. *Public Health.* 110: 331–8.
2 Department of Health (1992) *Health of the Nation: a strategy for health in England.* Cmd 1986. HMSO, London.
3 Department of Health (1999) *Saving Lives: our healthier nation.* Cmd 4386. The Stationery Office, London.

4   Department of Health (1997) *The New NHS: modern, dependable.* Cmd
    3807. The Stationery Office, London.
5   Goldblatt P (ed) (1990) *Longitudinal Study: mortality and social organ-
    isation, 1971–1981.* OPCS Series No. 6. HMSO, London.
6   Kendrick S and Clarke J (1993) The Scottish record linkage system.
    Health Bulletin. **51**(2): 72–9.
7   Herman AA, McCarthy BJ, Bakewell JM *et al.* (1997) Data linkage
    methods used in maternally-linked birth and infant death surveillance
    datasets from the United States (Georgia, Missouri, Utah and
    Washington State), Israel, Norway, Scotland and Western Australia.
    Paediatric and Perinatal Epidemiology. **11** (Suppl): 5–22.
8   Sorock GS, Smith GS, Reeve GR *et al.* (1997) Three perspectives on
    work-related injury surveillance systems. *American Journal of Industrial
    Medicine.* **32**: 116–28.
9   Dawson C, Perkins M, Draper E *et al.* (1997) Are outcome data
    regarding the survivors of neonatal care available from routine
    sources? *Archives of Diseases in Childhood.* **77**: F206–10.
10 Godden S and Pollock AM (1998) How to profile the population's
    use of health care and social care in one district. *Journal of Public Health
    Medicine.* **20**: 175–9.
11 Gissler M, Hemminki E, Louhiala P *et al.* (1998) Health registers as a
    feasible means of measuring health status in childhood – a 7-year
    follow-up of the 1987 Finnish birth cohort. *Paediatric and Perinatal
    Epidemiology.* **12**: 437–55.
12 Alsop JC and Langley JD (1998) Determining first admissions in a
    hospital discharge file via record linkage. *Methods of Information in
    Medicine.* **37**: 32–7.
13 Waller JA (1985) *Injury Control: a guide to the causes and prevention of
    trauma.* Lexington Books, Lexington, MA.
14 Haddon W (1980) Advances in the epidemiology of injuries as a basis
    for public health policy. *Public Health Reports.* **95**: 411–21.
15 Public Health Information Strategy Project Team (1993) *Improving
    Information on Accidents.* Public Health Information Strategy Imple-
    mentation Project 19. Department of Health, London.
16 Public Health Information Strategy Project Team (1996) *Agreeing an
    Accident Information Structure.* Public Health Information Strategy
    Implementation Project 19B. Department of Health, London.
17 Cryer PC, Jarvis SN, Edwards P *et al.* (1999) *How Can We Reliably
    Measure the Occurrence of Non-fatal Injury?* South East Institute of Public
    Health, Tunbridge Wells.
18 Haigney D (1995) STATS 19. *The Journal of the Institute of Road Safety
    Officers.* October: 11–17.

19 Health and Safety Executive (1992) *Reporting under RIDDOR.* Health and Safety Executive, Sheffield.

20 Health and Safety Executive (1985) *A Guide to the Reporting of Injuries, Diseases and Dangerous Occurrences Regulations 1985.* HS(R)23. The Stationery Office, London.

21 Stevens G (1992) Workplace injury: a view from the HSE's trailer to the 1990 Labour Force Survey. *Employment Gazette.* December: 621–38.

22 Newcombe HB (1988) *Handbook of Record Linkage: methods of health and statistical studies, administration, and business.* Oxford University Press, Oxford.

23 Jaro MA (1995) Probabilistic linkage of large public health data files. *Statistics in Medicine.* **14**: 491–8.

24 Cryer C, Brunning D and Rahman M (1995) *Injury Prevention Through Data Linkage. Phase 2: Data linkage pilot. The linkage of police road traffic accident reports to hospital admissions in East Sussex.* South East Institute of Public Health, Tunbridge Wells.

25 Austin KP (1992) A linked police and hospital database for Humberside. *Traffic Engineering and Control.* **33**: 674–83.

26 Nicholl JP (1984) *The Use of Hospital Inpatient Data in the Analysis of the Injuries Sustained by Road Accident Casualties.* TRRL Supplementary Report 628. Transport and Road Research Laboratory, Crowthorne.

27 Stone RD (1984) *Computer Linkage of Transport and Health Data.* TRRL Laboratory Report 1130. Transport and Road Research Laboratory, Crowthorne.

28 NHS Executive CRIR Secretariat (1997) *NHS Data Manual. Version 5.0.* NHS Executive, Leeds.

29 James HF (1991) Under-reporting of road traffic accidents. *Traffic Engineering and Control.* **32**: 574–83.

12 Statistical returns: past, present and future

Vic Kempner

Introduction

Throughout the first 50 years of the NHS there has been an unremitting preoccupation with trying to measure what it does and what it achieves. This is not really surprising as the NHS remains a politically sensitive, multi-billion pound enterprise. It operates 24 hours a day, 7 days a week and 52 weeks of the year, is among the largest employers in the UK, and touches every member of the population. There can be few multinational conglomerates equalling its complexity. Whilst it is unlikely that such interest in measurement will diminish during the next 50 years, there remains a need to continue the movement from a blunderbuss 'if it moves, then count it' philosophy towards something more focused and directed.

The phrase 'statistical returns' – or more commonly, 'central returns' – has generally come to be accepted as a term embracing the whole range of routine submissions of aggregate activity data. The information from central returns is seen as essential to the Department of Health for performance management, securing and allocating resources and policy formulation. In the Health Services Circular HSC 1999/070 the Department defines them as a structured collection of data from the NHS that they commission. Regional offices of the NHS Executive are included in this commissioning process.[1]

HSC 1999/070, referred to above, also lists each statistical return required by the Department of Health with the rationale for their being required. An updated circular is normally published every April and sent to all NHS trusts and health authorities; it is also available on the Department's website (http://www.open.gov.uk/doh/outlook.htm).

Some returns cover counts of events about patients – for example, the number of consultant outpatient attendances in general surgery in a particular trust. Others are concerned with rates about patients, such as the immunisation rate for measles, mumps and rubella in a particular health authority area. These counts and rates are not submitted as data about individual patients; this type of information is covered in Chapter 4 on Hospital Episode Statistics (HES).

The submissions are made predominantly to the Department of Health/NHS Executive. A limited number are made to other government departments or agencies. The annual submission on injuries resulting from fireworks is made to the Department for Trade and Industry. Central returns are made at varying intervals, some being monthly or quarterly and others being annual for the financial year (April to March).

For the sake of completeness, mention must be made of the various other returns which cover work force, ambulance transport, estates and finance. These are not specifically covered in this chapter.

Because returns are made at the level of trust, health authority and general practice there is a need for consistent counting. The *NHS Data Dictionary* contains definitions of all of the terms used, whilst the *NHS Data Manual* includes descriptions of how data items described in the Data Dictionary are used to derive the information for central returns. Changes to central information requirements are notified through *Data Set Change Notices* (DSCNs). These three sets of documentation are issued on disk to NHS trusts and health authorities by the NHS Information Authority.

Central returns are controlled through the Review of Central Returns Steering Committee (ROCR). The membership of ROCR is largely from the Department of Health and NHS Executive, but it does also have NHS trust members. Details of, and consultation on, new returns and changes to existing ones are discussed with the service through NHS representatives on the Committee for Regulating Information Requirements (CRIR). *Inter alia,* CRIR considers the burden that data collection for central returns will have on the NHS, and examines the impact that changes to data requirements will have on information systems. Although there is a long-established understanding that the service will normally be given 6 months notice of changes which have a significant impact on systems, there have been occasions when the notice period has been much shorter.

Looking back

The existence of central returns is certainly not new. The general direction for meeting central information requirements was established at the outset of the NHS, and conceptually the change since then has been remarkably small. This is quite helpful in allowing some high level historical comparisons to be made. The 300-page compendium of hospital statistics for 1949[2] provides some interesting browsing.

In 1949 the largest institution was Whittingham Hospital near Preston, which was classified as a mental hospital. It had a bed availability on 31 December 1949 of 3038 but an average daily bed occupation for the year of 3176. The inference is that temporary extra beds were brought into use on a regular basis. Data quality was clearly a problem then as now, since there are no figures provided for medical staffing levels.

In England and Wales, the total bed allocation in 1949 was 468 771. Of these, 42% were classified as beds for mental illness and mental deficiency, with a further 11% classified as tuberculosis and infectious diseases. Some of the latter beds were in institutions such as Clandon Smallpox Hospital and Tunbridge Wells Isolation Hospital.

The form in which the data are presented limits the type of calculations that can be done. It is interesting that Morriston Hospital, Swansea – the largest maternity type hospital (defined as 'Admitting only maternity cases') with a complement of 450 beds – had an average length of stay of 27.5 days. The hospital's midwifery staff numbered ten full time and two part-time.

Essentially, the need for data to be submitted to the Ministry of Health to meet its requirements for public accountability through Parliament in 1949 is little changed in terms of the Department of Health today and the central management role of the NHS Executive. The healthcare agenda is wider and more complex, the understanding of interrelationships between inputs and outputs is better (in some areas at least) and the demand has grown for more and better information both within the NHS and from the public.

Körner

Until the review chaired by Mrs Körner in the early 1980s[3] there had been considerable stability among central returns. Key forms, such as the annual hospital return SH3, had remained remarkably similar year on year thus allowing time series to be constructed with relative ease. The drawback, however, was the limited extent of definitions and the variability of their interpretation. The numbers of staff whose main role was to prepare, interpret and use information was very limited, and they generally resided only in the major teaching hospitals and regional hospital boards.

Edith Körner's review of NHS information marked a significant turning point in central returns as well as other areas of information around non-aggregated data. For the first time in an overt way the starting point was to talk about the business of the NHS and then construct the data needed to support the business functions. Another key principle was that if a particular piece of information was not needed at the operational level then it was unlikely to be required further up the NHS hierarchy at region or department level.

There was also a clear view that management information should be generated as a by-product of a clinical operational process and not be made an additional burden or overhead. This sentiment remains very valid but is still far from being a totally realised ambition.

Although the basis of the Körner principles was not new, this was the first time that a national review of information had been set up and was making very positive statements about the philosophy of information flows. Inevitably, the road to hell is paved with good intentions and unfortunately, what the Steering Group intended to be interim solutions were made permanent and their intended subsequent work was thwarted.[4] Thus, over time some 'Körnerisms' began to be diluted, only to be resurrected almost two decades later in the 1998 information strategy, *Information for Health*.[5]

In a number of respects the Körner review started a new chapter. Some of the pre-Körner returns became obsolete, others were modified and a whole tranche of new ones appeared. New concepts in recording and counting activities and events were introduced and old ones had to be forgotten. Principal among the new concepts was that of the minimum data set, whilst events such as hospital discharges and deaths were superseded by consultant episodes and provider spells. There was also an aim that an increasing amount of recording would be undertaken by clinical staff. Taken together, this meant that a comprehensive set of definitions had to be produced so that the larger number of staff involved in recording data as a normal part of their work would be doing so on a consistent basis.

One problem of the early post-Körner scene was the inevitable settling down period during which the quality of data was questionable. A further one was the move from the traditional calendar year to the financial year, which led to a 15-month period with effectively no or limited information. Once the new regime was underway the inevitable break in time series had to be overcome, and although some pre- and post-Körner comparisons were possible, there was a period of relative statistical famine.

On reflection, the Körner statistical revolution probably remains the single most important event in the first 50 years of NHS information and will influence thinking at the start of the new millennium. It raised the profile of information but perhaps more importantly, for the first time took a corporate rather than piecemeal look at the needs of the service, ending the separation of data for local and central requirements.[6] The name of Dame Edith Körner has become as much part of NHS jargon as is a minimum data set or a face-to-face contact.

Information

Körner as a sentinel event of the 1980s has already been mentioned, but there was actually another watershed event for health data in the previous decade which could easily be missed by the casual observer. This was the emergence of a new breed of technician called the information officer sometime in the 1970s. Quite soon, no self-respecting health organisation would be seen without its information officer whose particular skills were in understanding what the data meant as well as analysing it. Previously, data had sat around rather like gravy on a plate, whilst now, some information officers introduced a zest to the gravy, and others added a sauce.

This information explosion probably began as a minor detonation in the mid-1970s with the emerging demands of the newly restructured and integrated NHS. On 1 April 1974 the previously separately managed streams of hospital, community and family practitioner services were brought together, and the service began to realise that it needed a different type of data if the evolving health agenda was going to be progressed and implemented. Until then, central returns were essentially characterised as a necessary evil whose contents had little relevance to running operational services. Indeed, the bottom–up pressure for improvement was important in ensuring the establishment and support for the Körner review.

Whilst today many central returns are still seen as a low priority, over the past two decades there has developed an increasing appreciation of the need for them. In addition, an awareness grew of the use to which they could be put locally so that they were not just seen as 'feeding the beast' centrally. This change in attitude has been facilitated by the gradual trend away from the Department of Health and NHS Executive merely producing annual compendia of national summaries of returns towards publishing value-added information to enable meaningful comparisons and benchmarkings to be undertaken.

The value of national summaries of central returns merely assembled from the individual submissions of trusts and other organisations, and published as reference volumes, should not be dismissed lightly. When brought together with other appropriate sources of health information, they provide a major resource to underpin research, planning, benchmarking, performance management, policy development, and many more areas of work requiring a quantitative foundation.

The use of central returns might be greater by those working within the NHS if access to them was easier without needing to re-key the data into spreadsheets or databases. Sadly these annual summaries are still published in hard copy format much as they were 50 years ago. Electronic dissemination on disk or CD or via the Department's website would be a helpful step forward.

Some innovative research by John Yates at the Health Services Management Centre, Birmingham, in the 1970s looked at formal enquiries into incidents against patients in mental illness and mental handicap hospitals, and their correlation with poor levels of staffing and facilities. This work made use of the wealth of information recorded on the annual central return of psychiatric facilities, form SBH112. The natural and concerning observation from this analysis is that this information had been collected for many years but previously had not been used in a proactive manner. This important piece of work led Yates to extend his area of research and later set up the Inter-Authority Comparative Analysis Service.

The Department's development programme for performance indicators (PIs), and latterly, health service indicators (HSIs) drew on the huge volumes of largely untouched data in the central returns (these were not the sole sources of data). This marked an important change of emphasis. The inevitable response of comparisons being odious unless really meaningful comparisons are made helped fuel a new cottage industry that looked at means of ensuring that apples were being compared with apples and not with pears. The use of standardisation and normalisation helped this progress; however, an appreciation among users outside the information fraternity that relative values rather than absolute values could have significant meanings took time to emerge.

Today, there is a wide range of comparative indicators, initially those developed to support the contracting process,[7] and those being evaluated for the agenda resulting from the current NHS White Paper.[8] Indicators do not solely rely on aggregated data from central returns but draw extensively on much of the material covered in other chapters. This is equally the case with the emerging tranche of clinical indicators,[9] and with information needed to support national service frameworks[10] and clinical governance.

Information for Health has been very clearly promoted as an information strategy and not as either an information technology or information management and technology strategy.[5] It is formed around the information requirements which derive from *The New NHS* and the various initiatives, guidance and policies which have followed from it. The direction is focused on the information needs of clinicians and information to support clinical processes, which interestingly is a view that emerged some 30 years earlier in the first Cogwheel report.[11]

Looking ahead

The significant impacts of *Information for Health* and its role in facilitating the broad health agenda will not become widely apparent until the early years of the third millennium. What effects might these have on statistical or central returns as we know them?

The further development of patient-based data around the electronic patient record (EPR) and electronic health record (EHR), together with increased exploitation of the NHS-wide Clearing Service (NWCS) and NHSnet (the NHS private wide area network), could mean that the aggregate central return becomes a thing of the past. As seen, for example, with HES data in Chapter 4, appropriately anonymised data about individual patients allow an infinite range of analysis and aggregation to be performed centrally to support departmental and other policy and decision processes. Extending the HES principle through other data sets is clearly feasible.

Central returns on facilities, such as diagnostic departments currently handled through the annual KH12, may not be replaced in the short term. Means should be developed so that many of them are superseded by more contemporary and less burdensome methods of providing the data. These new means may also lead to improvements in the accuracy and integrity of the data.

L'envoi

Looking back over 50 years of statistical returns shows that although significant changes have occurred, conceptually they remain much the same. What about the next 50 years? Will there be counts of telecare contacts or rates of consultation in virtual hospitals? The due processes of effective service management and political accountability, hopefully accompanied increasingly by outcome and effectiveness studies, will remain to be fuelled. This should increasingly also provide information to be used advantageously by clinicians and managers at all levels. The only certainty is that statistical returns will still be around in some form or other.

References

1 Department of Health (1999) *Central Data Collections from the NHS.* Health Service Circular HSC 1999/070. DoH, London.

2 National Health Service (1952) *Hospital and Specialist Services, England and Wales: statistics for the year ended 31st December 1949.* HMSO, London.

3 Department of Health and Social Security Steering Group on Health Services Information (1982) *First Report to the Secretary of State.* HMSO, London.

4 Rigby M (1998) Information in child health management. In: Rigby M, Ross EM and Begg NT (eds) *Management for Child Health.* Chapman and Hall, London.

5 NHS Executive (1998) *Information for Health: an information strategy for*

the modern NHS 1998–2005: a national strategy for local implementation. Health Service Circular HSC 98/168. NHSE, Leeds.

6   Windsor P (1986) *Introducing Körner.* British Journal of Healthcare Computing Publications, Sutton.

7   Department of Health (1989) *Working for Patients.* Cmd 555. HMSO, London.

8   Department of Health (1997) *The New NHS: modern, dependable.* Cmd 3807. The Stationery Office, London.

9   Department of Health (1999) *Improving Quality and Performance in the New NHS: clinical indicators and high level performance indicators.* Health Service Circular HSC 1999/139. DoH, London.

10 Department of Health (1998) *National Service Frameworks.* Health Service Circular HSC 1998/074. DoH, London.

11 Ministry of Health (1967) *First Report of the Joint Working Party on the Organisation of Medical Work in Hospitals.* HMSO, London

Index

The New NHS: modern, dependable (1997 White Paper) 70, 71, 166, 176
NHS *see* National Health Service
NHS and Community Care Act, 1990 71
NHS Data Dictionary 192
NHS Data Manual 192
NHSnet 197–8
NHS Performance Assessment Framework (1999) 108
  mapping indicators to 128, 129–30
NHS Primary Care Act, 1997 71
NHS Trusts 58
  cancer data for 164–5
  see also hospitals
Nightingale, Florence 145
Northern Ireland 4–5, 134, 148, 152
  birth and maternity data 133, 137, 139, 143–4, 147
  child health system 144
Northern Ireland Office 5
Northern Ireland Statistics and Research Agency (NISRA) 134
Notification of Births Extension Act, 1915 141

obesity 86
occupation, parents' 135
occupational risks 42, 167
odds ratio 32
Office for National Statistics (ONS) 6–7, 134
  abortion data 39
  Advisory Groups 8
  births and maternity data 134, 137–8, 143, 151–2
  cancer data 37–8, 154–5, 166
  censuses and population estimates 35–6, 73–4
  congenital anomalies 38
  definitions used 27–33
  general practice records 39–41, 63–4
  health data (non-mortality) 35–50
  infectious diseases 37
  linked routinely collected data 41–2
  Longitudinal Study 41–2
  mortality data 13–26
  survey data 42–5
  syntheses of survey/other health data 45
  website 9
Office of Population, Censuses and Surveys (OPCS) 14, 134

see also Office for National Statistics
official statistics
  data quality 7
  data sources 6–7
  definition 1–2
  on Internet 6–7
  national coverage 4–5
  non-NHS sources 7–10
  users 5–6
  websites 2
older people
  falls in 178
  surveys of health 44, 85, 97
Omnibus Survey, ONS 43
ONS *see* Office for National Statistics
Open Government provisions 61
oral health 125
Our Healthier Nation (1998 consultative document) 72, 97, 100
outcomes, clinical and health *see* clinical and health outcomes
outpatient referrals 75
Oxford Cancer Information Unit 163
Oxford Record Linkage Study 23, 42, 128

parity 135
Patient Episode Data for Wales (PEDW) 147
patients
  experience 108
  Hospital Episode Statistics, *see* Hospital Episode Statistics
  individual records 61
  registration 67
  statistical returns 191–2
  surveys of NHS 70–1
Patients' Charter and You (1995) 156
PCGs *see* primary care groups
People Aged 65 and Over 44, 85
performance indicators (PIs) 197
  see also clinical and health outcomes and health indicators
perinatal mortality 139
period effects 27
pharmaceutical data 68–70
pharmacies, community 68, 70
poisoning, mortality data 17, 21, 22, 24
police
  data confidentiality issues 184
  road traffic accident data 175, 182–3, 186–8